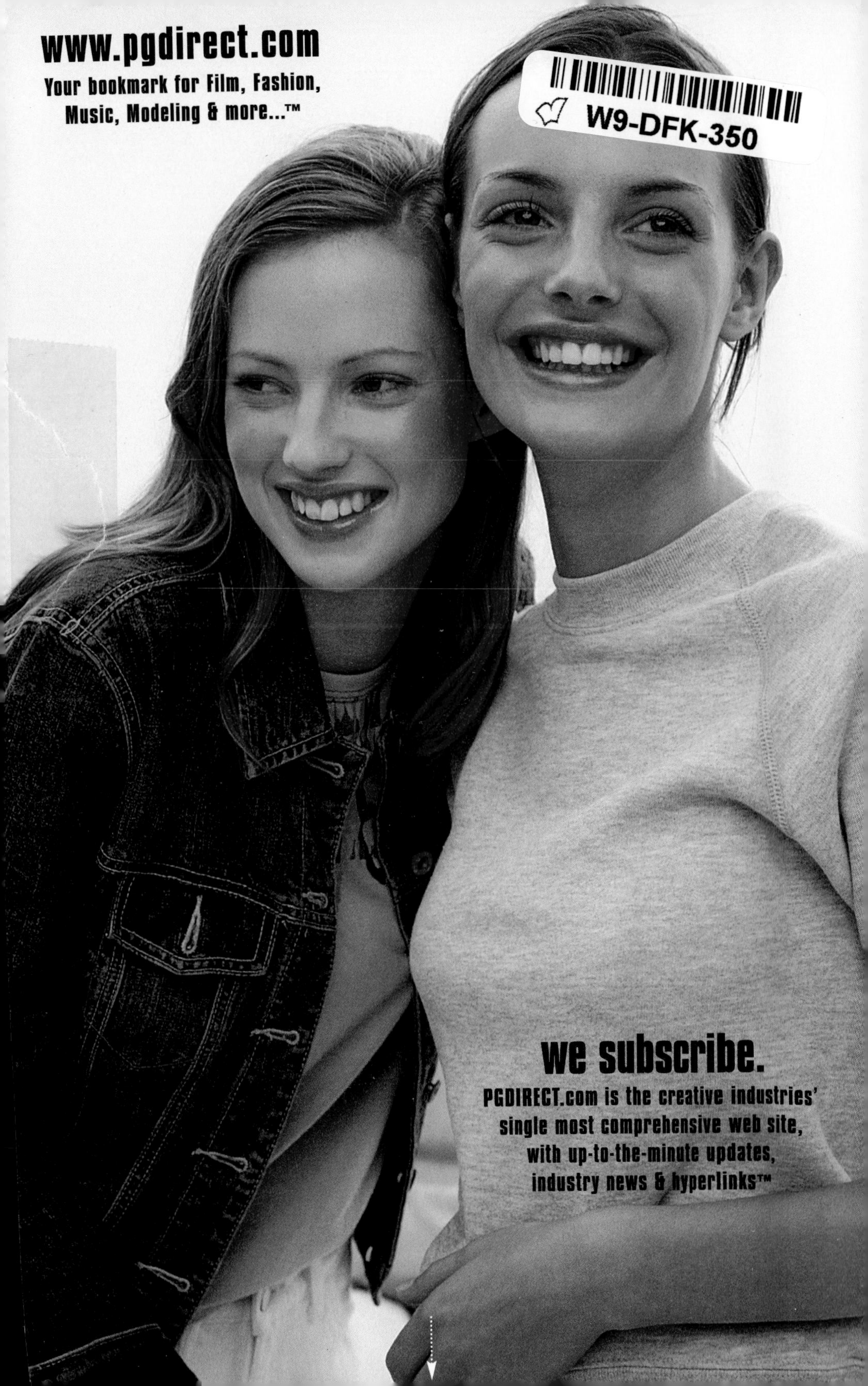
www.pgdirect.com
Your bookmark for Film, Fashion, Music, Modeling & more...™
we subscribe.
PGDIRECT.com is the creative industries' single most comprehensive web site, with up-to-the-minute updates, industry news & hyperlinks™

www.pgdirect.com

President/Publisher:
Gregory James

Vice President of Sales & Marketing:
Tricia Mazzilli-Blount

Directors:
Lawrence Brill
Umberto Guido III

Editor:
Jean Walkinshaw

Associate Editors:
Nina Smith
Diane Walkinshaw
Nancy Wojochowski

Database Consultant:
Debbra Lupien
Lupien Limited

Art Director:
Carol Petro
All Caps

Webmasters:
Jeff Friedman
Brian Mishico
Tim Mishico
Peter Rice
Barry Sergeant

Accountant:
Robert Vogler
RWV Management Corporation

Bookkeeper:
Margery Festini Kozdeba
MFK Management

Licensing Company:
Christine Annechino
ACA/The Licensing Group

Product Placement Agency:
Patti Ganguzza
AIM Productions Inc

Corporate Legal Sounsel:
William Barrett
Gary Young
Mandelbaum Salsburg

Copyright Legal Counsel:
Richard Klar
Richard Klar & Associates

Book Sales Distribution:
SCB Distributors
310.532.9400

Printing by
Offset Impressions, Inc.
www.offsetimpress.com
Printed in the USA

The Model & Talent 2001 is available for bulk orders or to advertise in the next edition of the Model & Talent 2002, contact:

Peter Glenn Publications
49 Riverside Avenue
Westport, CT 06880 USA
T: 203.227.4949
F: 203.227.6170
E: m&t2002@pgdirect.com

Early Reservation Deadline:
May 31st, 2001
Final Reservation Deadline:
September 28th, 2001

You can now personally update your listing information at any time via our web site.
Update area is found at:
www.pgdirect.com/update.

ISBN: 0-87314-144-X
$29.95

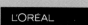

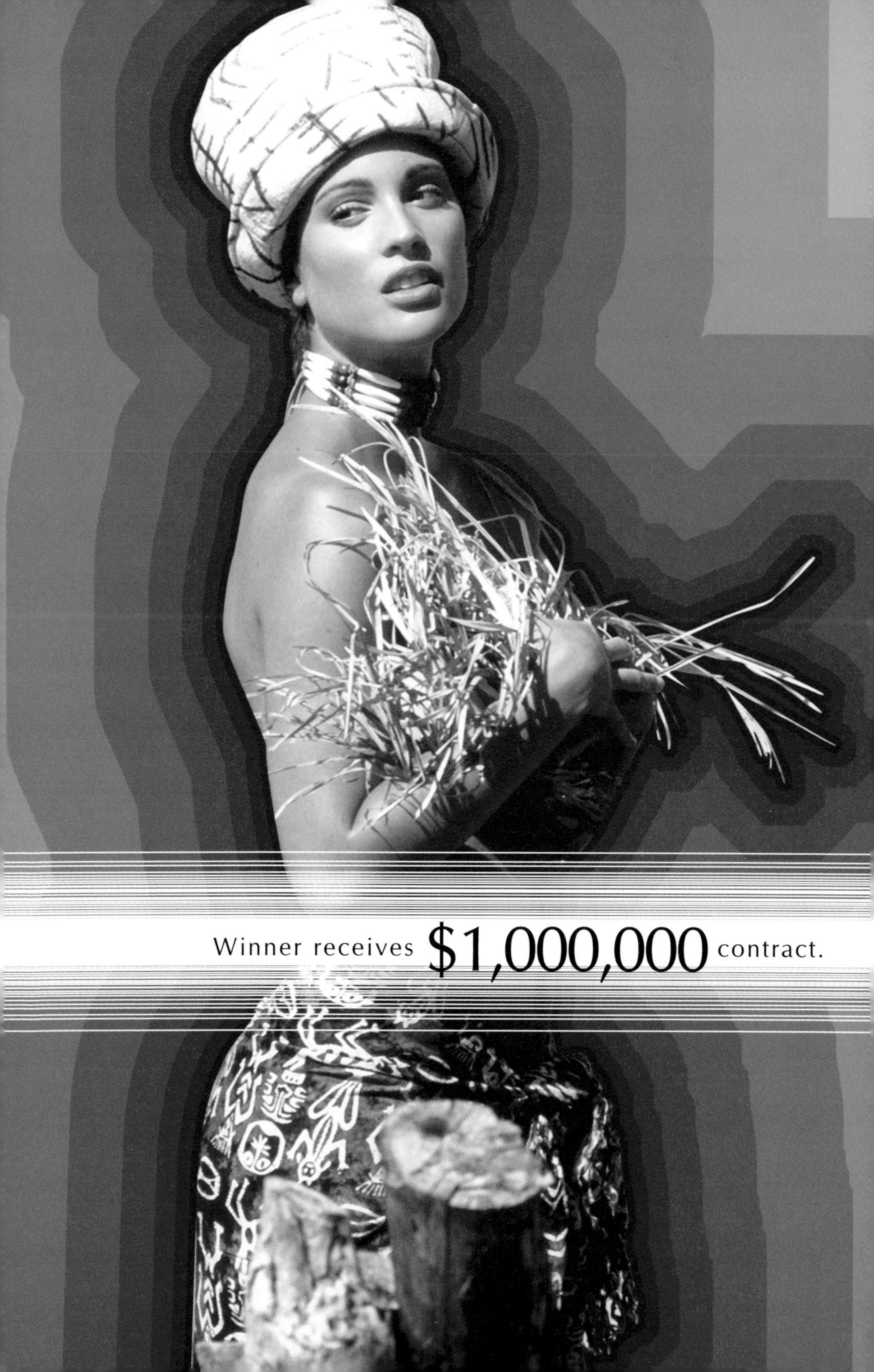
Winner receives $1,000,000 contract.

49 Riverside Avenue
Westport, Connecticut 06880

• • • •

T 1 203 227 4949
TF 1 888 332 6700
F 1 203 227 6170
E INFO@PGDIRECT.COM

Friends,

It is always important to remember that what the future offers us, the past has given us. Technology has provided us with ever-improving tools to accomplish our means and new generations of professionals will maximize the capacities of these innovations.

It is 10 years since the founder of PGP, Peter Glenn, passed. It was his innovation that fostered the dissemination of industry-wide information with the famous Madison Avenue Handbook. No publication provided more comprehensive, up-to-date information and no publisher was more respected for those efforts. Companies and individuals that represented the highest standards were included within the pages of the Handbook, and Peter and his staff kept a close eye on the inclusions. The integrity of the publication was defined by the integrity of those who were listed. The longevity of the businesses listed were testament to Peter's unfailing vigilance and genuine eye for talented, responsible professionals.

Some things don't change.

Almost 50 years since the inauguration of the Handbook, the same premises remain intact for Peter Glenn Publications and our web site, www.pgdirect.com. While the way we disseminate the information has changed somewhat, the criteria for inclusion has not altered one iota. We like to think that Mr. Glenn would be quite proud.

In the decade since Peter died much has, certainly, changed. Print, video, cable, internet have all expanded the way we see, hear and understand the world. Our industry, in large part, has been the recipient of this media largess. It is, however, the truly dedicated and enormously talented professionals that drive the continued growth. We celebrate those individuals by understanding and appreciating their accomplishments.

So, as the present dictates our future, we memorialize the past. As with Peter and his legacy, we remember and appreciate the valuable, remarkable contributions of those who have also left us. These contributions are not merely palpable, they are indelible.

The marvelous abilities of those who preceded us will only live on and prompt us to continue to achieve. To paraphrase, what the past has given, the future offers.

Most sincerely,

The Partners of Peter Glenn Publications

Gregory James President	Tricia Mazzilli-Blount Vice President	L. Chip Brill Director	Umberto Guido III Director

The Model & Talent 2001 Directory
is dedicated to the memory and accomplishments
of those who led the way before us.

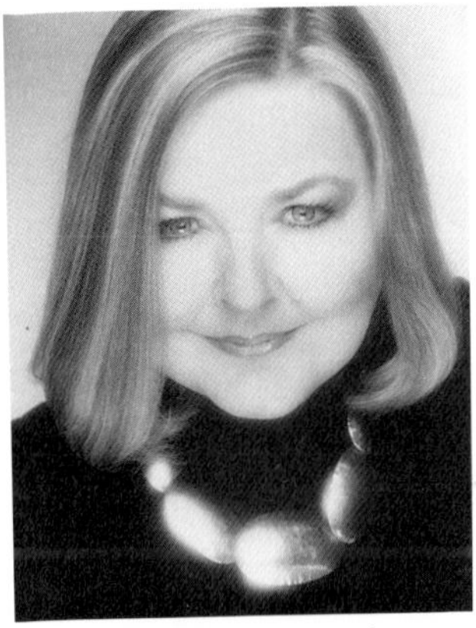

Dott Burns
1936–2000

Dorothy "Dott" Burns, the powerhouse talent agent died on April 31st at age 64. Dott was known for having a velvet fist in an iron glove, she once said "Keep your clothes on and a smile on your face."

Dott will long be remembered for her some thirty years of service and the launching of countless careers. Burn's talent have appeared in scores of commercials and television programs such as *Leave it To Beaver, America's Most Wanted*, and *Miami Vice* as well as movies such as *Smokey and The Bandit, GI Jane* and, *Great Expectations.*

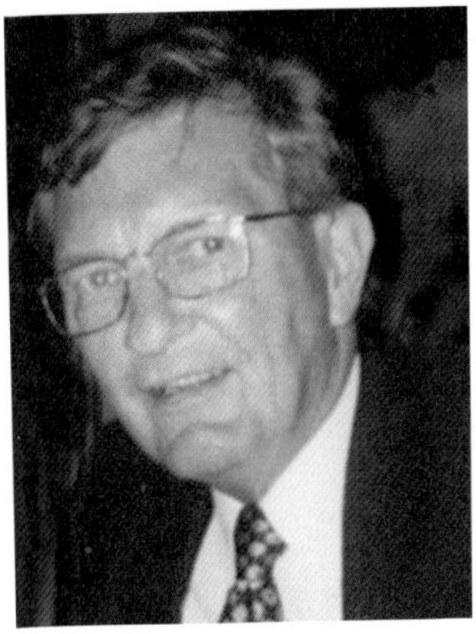

Ken Johnson
1929–2000

Ken Johnson, a well respected architect died on June 22nd at age 70. After retiring in 1988 from his successful architectural firm, ISD, Ken joined his wife & life-long partner in running the prestigious Susanne Johnson Talent Agency in Chicago and with him brought the spirit and guidance from his architectural days to the modeling industry.

Ken had these words to say, "Have fun, enjoy yourself. Remember that you're building something that is lasting - and do it with honesty and imagination." Good words of advice for any business or industry.

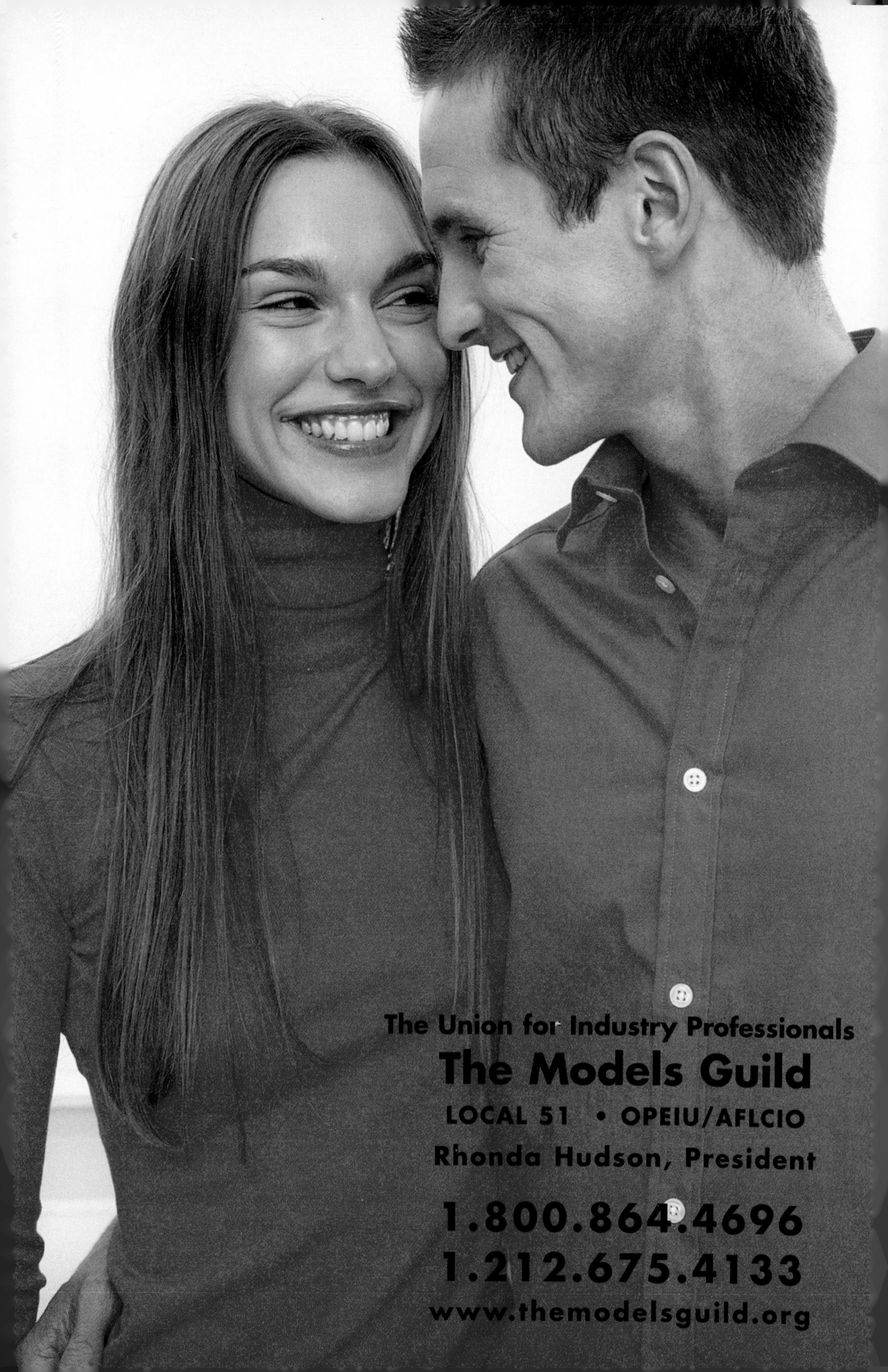
The Union for Industry Professionals
The Models Guild
LOCAL 51 • OPEIU/AFLCIO
Rhonda Hudson, President
1.800.864.4696
1.212.675.4133
www.themodelsguild.org

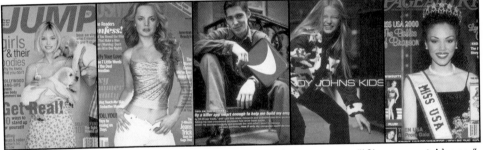

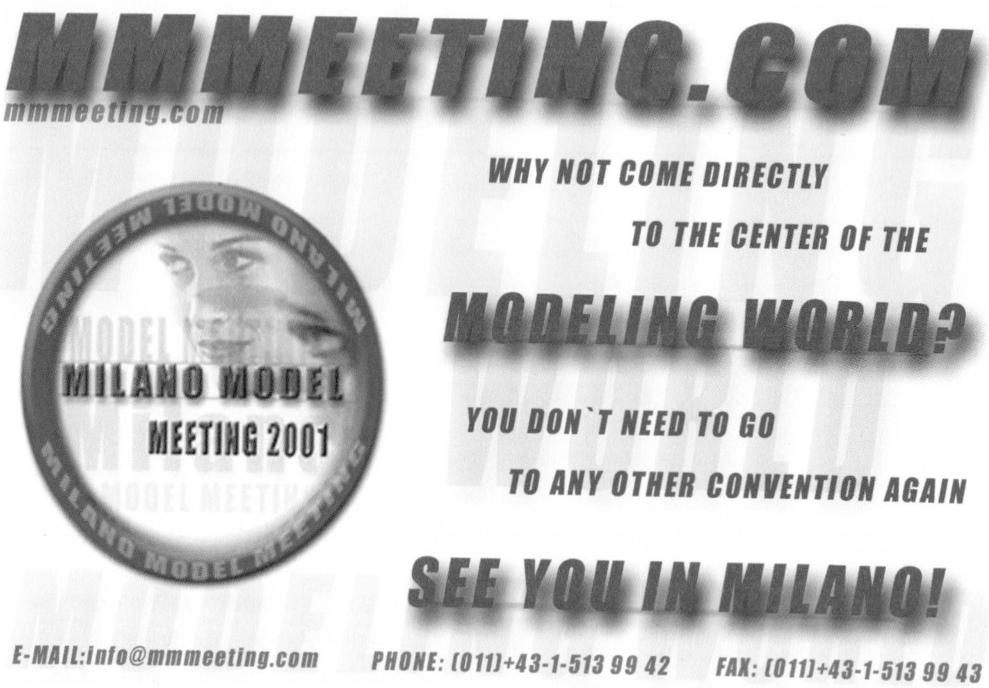

AGENCY BOOKS

F-SQUARED PRINTING
234 Fifth Aveunue, 4th Floor
New York, NY 10010 USA
T 1 888 652 9951
*See Ad Under Illinois & Texas Sections.

ASSOCIATIONS/COMPETITIONS FOR THE MODELING INDUSTRY

AMERICAN MODELING & TALENT COMPETITION • AMTC
510 Haddington Lane
Peachtree City, GA 30269 USA
Contact: Carey Lewis Arban
T 1 770 487 6656
F 1 770 487 6763
W www.mlamtc.com
E warban@mindspring.com
*See Ad This Section.

AMERICAN TALENT SHOWCASE
141 Gadesen Street
Chester, SC 29706 USA
Contact: Donna Ehrlich
T 1 803 581 2278
F 1 803 581 7703
W www.oneats.com

ASSOCIATIONS/COMPETITIONS

CANADIAN MODEL & TALENT CONVENTION
291 Front Street
Belleville, ON K8N 2Z6 Canada
Contact: Audra Anderson
T 1 613 967 5972
F 1 613 967 1544
E cmtc.inc@sympatico.ca

CONNECTIONS MODEL & TALENT CONVENTION
12638-16 Jefferson Avenue
Contact: Pat Wright
Newport News, VA 23602 USA
T 1 757 877 4150
F 1 757 886 9128

Elite's "Look of the Year"
111 E 22nd Street
New York, NY 10010 USA
T 1 212 529 9700

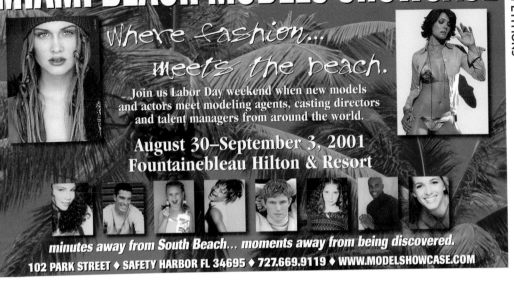

Faces West International Model & Talent Convention
212-1008 Homer Street
Vancouver, BC V6B 2X1 Canada
T 1 604 683 5536
F 1 604 228 4039

Ford's "Supermodel of the World" Contest
142 Greene Street
New York, NY 10012 USA
T 1 212 219 7020
F 1 212 966 5028

International Model & Talent Association
2525 E Camelback Road
Phoenix, AZ 85016 USA
T 1 602 954 1390
F 1 602 954 1393

MB MODEL & TALENT EXPO
624 W University Drive, Suite 180
Denton, TX 76201 USA
Contact: Mike Beaty
T 1 940 243 2222
F 1 940 243 2225
W www.mbexpo.com

MIAMI BEACH MODELS SHOWCASE
102 Park Street
Safety Harbor, FL 34695 USA
Contact: Pamela Osler-Oleck & Suzan Speer
T 1 727 669 9119
F 1 727 669 6217
W www.modelshowcase.com
E MBMSHOW@aol.com
***See Ad This Section**

MISS AMERICA ORGANIZATION
2 Ocean Way, Suite 1000
Atlantic City, NJ 08401 USA
T 1 609 345 7571
F 1 609 347 6079

MMMEETING.COM • MILANO MODEL MEETING
T 43 1 513 99 42
F 43 1 513 99 43
W www.mmmeeting.com
E info@mmmeeting.com
***See Ad This Section**

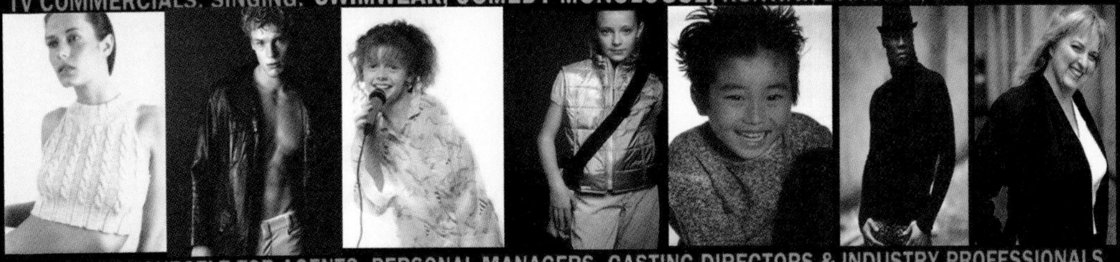

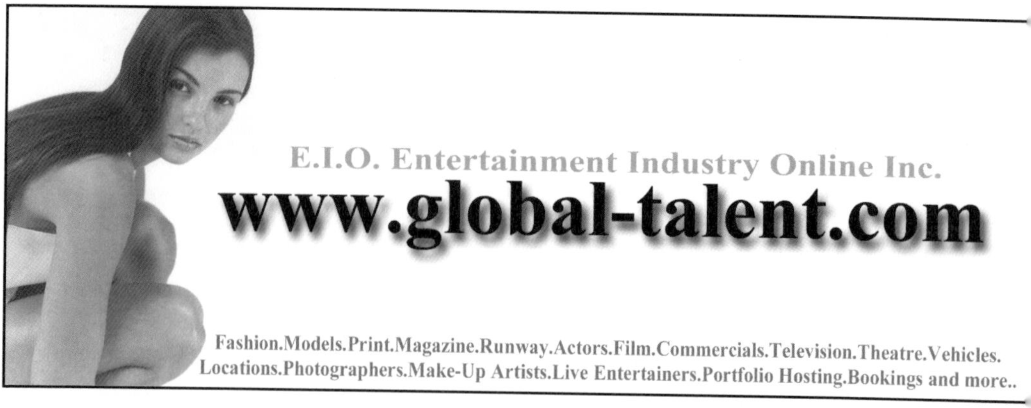

MODEL MAKERS INTERNATIONAL
P.O. Box 11117
Jackson, TN 38308 USA
Contact: Darla Caldwell, President
T 1 731 664 9647
F 1 731 660 5907
W www.modelmakersinternational.com
E modelmakersintl@aol.com
*See Ad This Section.

MODELING ASSOCIATION OF AMERICA INTERNATIONAL INC
951 Doyle Street
Orangeburg, SC 29115 USA
Contact: Betty Lane Gramling, Membership Chair
A Not-for-Profit Corporation.
T 1 803 534 9672
T 1 212 753 1555 MAAI in NY
F 1 803 535 3000
W www.maai.org

MODELS OF THE SOUTH
907 Beveridge Road
Richmond, VA 23226 USA
Contact: Jack Rasnic
T 1 804 285 8450
F 1 804 288 7024

Modeling Association of Canada
176 Rupert Street
Thunder Bay, ON P7B 3X1 Canada
T 1 807 345 2126
F 1 807 346 0915

PAC • THE PERFORMING ARTS CHAMPIONSHIP
P.O. Box 750
Seattle, WA 98101-0750 USA
Contact: Sunny Chae
T 1 206 467 4974
F 1 206 467 4976
*See Ad This Section.

RUNWAY TO SUCCESS
1519 N 23rd Street, Suite 203
Wilmington, NC 28405 USA
Contact: Delia Harper
T 1 910 343 1753
T 1 910 343 0690
F 1 910 343 9473
E DMMMDLS@aol.com
*See Ad This Section.

WORLDWIDE MODEL & TALENT CONVENTION
Mission Square 16, 2901 University Avenue
Columbus, GA 31907 USA
T 1 706 561 9449
F 1 706 561 9741

ATTORNEYS: ENTERTAINMENT

MICHAEL WALKER, P.A.
407 Lincoln Road, Suite 4E
Miami Beach, FL 33139 USA
T 1 305 531 5200
F 1 305 531 5206
E SoBeAtty@aol.com
*See Ad Under New York Section.

CASTING / WORLD WIDE WEB

E.I.O • ENTERTAINMENT INDUSTRY ONLINE INC
180-1027 Davie Street
Vancouver BC V6E 4L2 Canada
T 1 604 669 7838
F 1 604 844 7807
W www.global-talent.com
E webmaster@global-talent.com
*See Ad This Section.

MODELSANDTALENT.COM
1311 Howe Street, Suite 200
Vancouver, BC V6Z 2P3 Canada
Contact: Vanessa M. Helmer
T 1 604 221 4080
F 1 604 221 4071
W www.modelsandtalent.com
E info@modelsandtalent.com

COMPOSITES

99 RIGHT DESIGN
174 Spadina Avenue, Suite 606
Toronto, ON M5T 2C2 Canada
Contact: Brian Dort
T 1 416 504 5027
F 1 416 504 4018
W www.99right.com
*See Ad This Section.

ADVANCED DIGITAL GRAPHICS
1 W 22nd Street
New York, NY 10010 USA
T 1 212 645 5300
F 1 212 727 8253
W www.adggraphics.com
*See Ad Under NYC Model Agencies.

BUNKER PRODUCTIONS
957 N Cole
Los Angeles, CA 90038 USA
T 1 323 463 1070
F 1 323 463 1077
*See Ad Under LA Model Agencies.

DIGICARD
P.O. Box 877
Ft. Washington, PA 19034 USA
Contact: Dave Male
T 1 215 542 0200 Ext. 403
F 1 215 542 7586
W www.digi-card.com
E dsm@netreach.net
*See Ad This Section.

IMPRESSION COLOR
820 Jill Court
East Meadow, NY 11554 USA
Contact: Harold Selinger
T 1 888 820 9096
T 1 516 481 6247
F 1 516 481 6247
W www.impressioncolor.com
*See Ad Under NYC Model Agencies.

LED ZED COMPOSITES
415 Linville
Westland, MI 48185 USA
Contact: Emin
T 1 734 467 9337
F 1 734 728 3521
*See Ad Under NYC Model Agencies.

MEDIA 3 STUDIOS
20024 Ballinger Way NE
Seattle, WA 98155 USA
Contact: John Potter
T 1 206 363 5473
F 1 206 362 1710
W www.media3studios.com
E m3@media3studios.com
*See Ad This Section.

MODEL COMP
1487 Stewarts Ferry Pike
Hermitage, TN 37076 USA
Contact: R. Tracy Fitzgerald
T 1 615 885 0080
F 1 615 889 7944
W www.model-comp.com
E americangraphics@home.com
*See Ad This Section.

MODERN POSTCARD
1675 Faraday Avenue
Carlsbad, CA 92008 USA
Full Color Promotional Cards
T 1 800 959 8365
F 1 760 431 1939
W www.modernpostcard.com
*See Ad Under NYC Model Agencies.

PICTURE PERFECT INTERNATIONAL
1218 Washington Avenue
Miami Beach, FL 33139 USA
Contact: Patrice Hallot
T 1 305 674 1011
F 1 305 674 7978
W www.pictureperfectintl.com
E phallot@pictureperfectintl.com
*See Ad Under NYC Model Agencies.

PICTURE PERFECT INTERNATIONAL
23 Rue D'antin
Paris, 75002 France
T 33 1 43 12 82 50
F 33 1 43 12 82 51
W www.pictureperfectintl.com
E phallot@pictureperfectintl.com
*See Ad Under NYC Model Agencies.

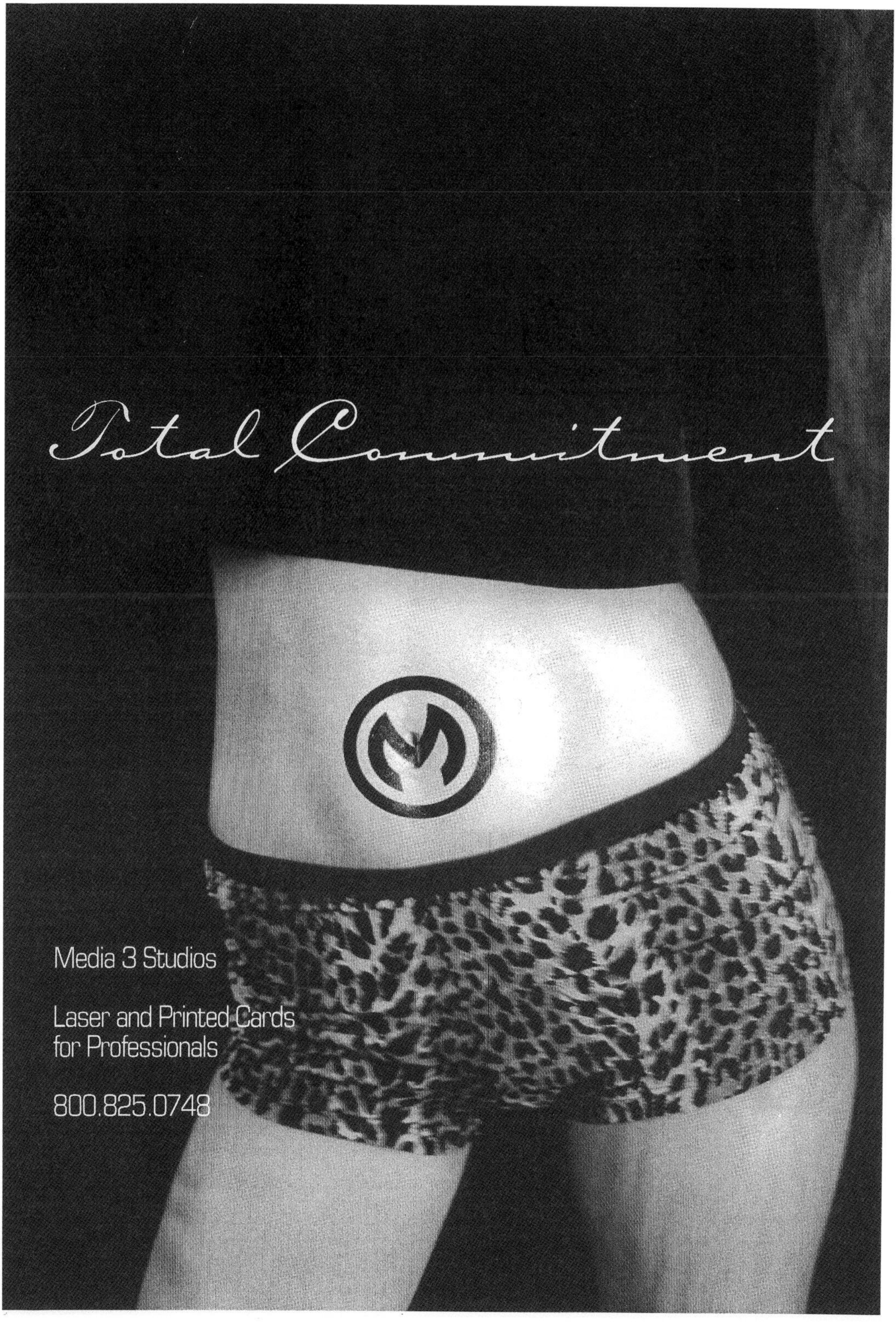
Total Commitment
Media 3 Studios
Laser and Printed Cards
for Professionals
800.825.0748

COMPOSITES

PRINT ON DEMAND BY BUNKER PRODUCTIONS
31 Union Square W, 2nd Floor
New York, NY 10003 USA
Contact: Michael Bunker, President
T 1 212 414 0317
F 1 212 414 0625
W www.printondemandnyc.com
*See Ad Under NYC Model Agencies.

COMPUTER SOFTWARE FOR THE INDUSTRY

CDS INC
270 Lafayette Street, Suite 1002
New York, NY 10012 USA
Contact: Susan Funk
Software solutions for booking,
picture management & scouting.
T 1 212 965 1193
F 1 212 965 1218

11x14.com
2677 Autumn Ridge Drive
Thousand Oaks, CA 91362 USA
Contact: Adam Pergament
Customized Websites, Internet Portfolios, Calendar
Booking Software...One Solution!
T 1 805 241 9979
F 1 805 492 4338
W www.11x14.com
*See Ad Under Los Angeles & New York Sections.

ORGANIZATIONS FOR THE MODELING INDUSTRY

MODELS FOR CHRIST
54 W 39th Street, 3rd Floor
New York, NY 10018 USA
T 1 212 780 4881
W www.modelsforchrist.com
E agents@modelsforchrist.com
*See Ad This Section.

THE MODELS GUILD
265 W 14th Street, Suite 203
New York, NY 10011 USA
Contact: Rhonda Hudson, President
T 1 800 864 4696
T 1 212 675 4133
W www.themodelsguild.org
*See Ad This Section.

PORTFOLIOS

PETER GLENN PUBLICATIONS
49 Riverside Avenue
Westport, CT 06880 USA
Contact: Gregory James
We carry heat-sealed vinyl & scuba portfolios
and now introducing our new Vienna line.
T 1 888 332 6700
T 1 203 227 4949
F 1 203 227 6170
W www.pgdirect.com

SCOUTING COMPANIES/ MODEL SEARCHES

LATIN SUPERMODEL SEARCH
1688 Meridian Avenue, Suite 801
Miami Beach, FL 33139 USA
T 1 305 604 8411
W www.latinsupermodelssearch.com
*See Ad This Section.

LOOKS WEST MODEL & TALENT SEARCH
3405 South Western, Suite 201
Amarillo, TX 79109 USA
Contact: Carol Henderson
T 1 806 352 1943
F 1 806 355 6154
W www.ModelsWest.com/LOOKSWEST
E modelswest@aol.com

MANHATTAN MODEL SEARCH
90 West Street, Suite 905
New York, NY 10006 USA
T 1 212 964 8274
F 1 212 964 7847

MODEL SEARCH AMERICA
588 Broadway, Suite 711
New York, NY 10012 USA
Contact: F. David Mogull, President
Linn Littland, Director of Model & Agent Relations
T 1 212 343 0100
F 1 212 966 3322
W www.supermodels.com
E msa@supermodels.com
*See Ad Under NYC Model Agencies.

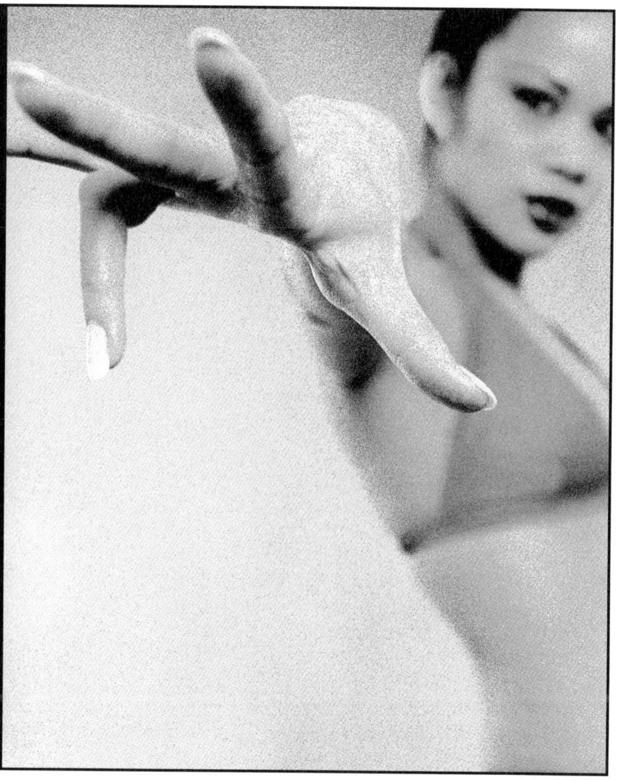

MODEL & TALENT SEARCH OF TEXAS
701 E Plano Parkway, Suite 409
Plano, TX 75074-6757 USA
Contact: Teresa Scordo, President
T 1 972 943 3334
F 1 972 943 3472
W www.modeltalentsearchoftx.com
E merina@modeltalentsearchoftx.com

WORLDWIDE MODEL GROUP
120 W Wieuca Road
Atlanta, GA 30342 USA
Contact: Jenifer Duggan
T 1 404 531 0030
F 1 404 459 8936
W www.worldwidemodelgroup.com

WEB DESIGN SERVICES FOR THE MODELING INDUSTRY

BEAUMONDE INC
1031 Beacon Street
Brookline, MA 02446 USA
Contact: Al Lakhina
T 1 800 894 3996
T 1 617 739 9803
F 1 617 739 9860
W www.beaumonde.com
E info@beaumonde.com
*See Ad on the Outside Back Cover.

11x14.com
2677 Autumn Ridge Drive
Thousand Oaks, CA 91362 USA
Contact: Adam Pergament
Customized Websites, Internet Portfolios, Calendar Booking Software...One Solution!
T 1 805 241 9979
F 1 805 492 4338
W www.11x14.com
*See Ad Under Los Angeles & New York Sections.

MODEL & TALENT AGENCIES

ALABAMA

Cathi Larsen Model & Talent Agency
1675 Mont Claire Road, Suite 136
Birmingham, AL 35210 USA
T 1 205 951 2445

E'LAN AGENCY
1446 Montgomery Highway
Birmingham, AL 35216 USA
Contact: Flora Price, President
T 1 205 823 9180
F 1 205 823 9177
W www.elanbirmingham.com
E elanagency@yahoo.com

Prater & Prater
2642 O'Neal Circle
Birmingham, AL 35226 USA
T 1 205 822 8135
F 1 205 979 0912

REAL PEOPLE MODELS & TALENT
714 32nd Street S
Birmingham, AL 35233 USA
Contact: Jay Brackin or Michael Fulmer
T 1 205 323 5437
F 1 205 323 3299
E agent@realpeople.com

PAMA AGENCY
708 Andrew Jackson Way
Huntsville, AL 35801 USA
Contact: Marie Hewett, Director
T 1 256 536 5200
F 1 256 536 5201
W www.pamamodels.com
E BVHewett@bellsouth.net

BAREFOOT MODELS & TALENT
750 Downtowner Loop W, Suite G
Mobile, AL 36609 USA
Contact: Suzanne Massingill
T 1 334 344 5554
F 1 334 344 3383
E barefootmodels@aol.com

CYNTHIA'S STUDIO MODEL & TALENT AGENCY
2030 4th Street E
Montgomery, AL 36106 USA
Contact: Cynthia or Bruce
T 1 334 272 5555
F 1 334 262 7616
E CynthiasTalent@aol.com

Macy's Modeling School
15 Choccolocca Street
Oxford, AL 36203 USA
T 1 256 835 5380

Talentscouts Model & Talent Management Company
5928 Shane Circle
Pinson, AL 35126 USA
T 1 205 681 5889
F 1 205 681 2891

Alabama Talent Management
P.O. Box 020198
Tuscaloosa, AL 35402-0198 USA
T 1 205 364 8700
F 1 205 364 8813

MODEL & TALENT AGENCIES

ALASKA

CUP'IK WARRIOR PRODUCTIONS
P.O. Box 110662
Anchorage, AK 99511-0662 USA
Contact: Grace Olrun, Vice President/Operations
T 1 907 258 2454
F 1 907 348 6681
W www.cupikwarrior.com
E cupik@cupikwarrior.com
***See Ad This Section.**

MODEL & TALENT AGENCIES

ARIZONA

Phoenix

Arizona Media Resources
4700 E Thomas Road, Suite 104
Phoenix, AZ 85018 USA
T 1 602 224 5888
F 1 602 957 4070

Dani's Agency
1 E Camelback Road, Suite 550
Phoenix, AZ 85012 USA
T 1 602 578 6837
F 1 602 277 7304

HPG AZ-TALENT
4747 N 7th Street, Suite 400
Phoenix, AZ 85014 USA
Contact: Joseph A. Herbert, Owner
T 1 602 263 8807
F 1 602 277 8790
W www.az-talent.com
E jahpc@msn.com

Jacquie Hughes Talent & Model Management/Casting
6209 N 21st Drive
Phoenix, AZ 85015-1902 USA
T 1 602 242 0306
F 1 602 265 1205

LEIGHTON AGENCY INC
2231 E Camelback Road, Suite 319
Phoenix, AZ 85016 USA
Contact: Ruth Leighton, President
SAG/AFTRA Franchised
T 1 602 224 9255
F 1 602 468 6888
W www.leightonagency.com

MODEL PLUS INTERNATIONAL
500 E Thomas Road, Suite 304
Phoenix, AZ 85019 USA
Contact: Pamela Young
T 1 602 234 2628
F 1 602 234 2788
W www.modelplusintl.com

SIGNATURE MODELS & TALENT
2600 North 44th Street, Suite 209
Phoenix, AZ 85008 USA
Broadcast Media/Print: Terri Hoffmann
T 1 480 966 1102
F 1 602 381 0956

THE YOUNG AGENCY
500 East Thomas Road, Suite 304
Phoenix, AZ 85012 USA
Contact: Pamela A. Young
T 1 602 212 2668
F 1 602 234 2788
W www.modelsplusintl.com
E modelsplus@earthlink.net

Scottsdale

ARIZONA MODELS & PROMOTIONS
4435 N Saddlebag Trail, Suite 3
Scottsdale, AZ 85251 USA
Contact: Dana Van Deman
T 1 480 994 0880
F 1 480 994 4748
W www.azmodels.com
E azmodlin@aol.com

ELIZABETH SAVAGE TALENT
4949 E Lincoln Drive
Scottsdale, AZ 85253 USA
Contact: Elizabeth Savage
T 1 602 840 3530
F: 1 602 840 7024

FORD ROBERT BLACK AGENCY
4300 North Miller Road, Suite 202
Scottsdale, AZ 85251 USA
Contact: Robert Black, President
T 1 480 966 2537
F 1 480 967 5424
E FORDRBA@aol.com

John Robert Powers
5225 N Scottsdale Road
Scottsdale, AZ 85250 USA
T 1 480 424 7287
F 1 480 947 5046

L'Image/John Casablancas
7426 E Stetson Drive, Suite 220
Scottsdale, AZ 85251 USA
T 1 480 941 4838
F 1 480 941 4856

>>

ARIZONA

NETWORK INTERNATIONAL INC
7025 East McDowell Road, Suite 1A
Scottsdale, AZ 85257 USA
Contact: Patrik Simpson / Royal Robins
T 1 480 941 6922
F 1 480 941 6933
W www.network-models.com
E NETWORKAZ@aol.com
***See Ad This Section.**

Tuscon

ACT THEATRICAL & MODELING AGENCY
3400 E Speedway, Suite 206
Tucson, AZ 85716 USA
Contact: Berenda Crellin, Director
T 1 520 795 4615
F 1 520 795 1935
W www.actmodelsactors.com
E actagy@azstar.com

BARBIZON OF TUCSON
4811 East Grant Road, Suite 255
Tucson, AZ 85712 USA
Contact: Melissa Isaak, Owner
or Wendy Franklin, Agency Director
T 1 520 323 5010
F 1 520 323 7797
W www.barbizonmodeling.com
E Barbmodels@aol.com

ELIZABETH SAVAGE TALENT
616 N Country Club Drive
Tucson, AZ 85716 USA
T 1 520 795 8585
F 1 520 795 5064

FLAIR / NETWORK INTERNATIONAL INC
6458 N Oracle Road, Suite 1
Tucson, AZ 85704 USA
Contact: Marie Sarkiss
T 1 520 742 1090
F 1 520 742 3809
W www.network-models.com
E NETWORKAZ@aol.com
***See Ad This Section.**

Fosi's Modeling & Talent Agency
2777 N Campbell, Suite 209
Tucson, AZ 85719 USA
T 1 520 795 3534
F 1 520 795 6037

TUCSON MODEL GROUP
8141 E Bellevue
Tucson, AZ 85715 USA
Contact: Janet Ryan
T 1 520 751 8312
F 1 520 751 8312
W www.tucsonmodelgroup.com
E tucsonmodelgroup@cs.com

ARKANSAS

MTM Agency/John Casablancas
416 West Meadow
Fayetteville, AR 72701 USA
T 1 501 444 7972
F 1 501 587 8555

Wings International Agency
478 CR 324
Jonesboro, AR 72401 USA
T 1 870 933 7400
F 1 870 933 7400

THE AGENCY INC
802 West 8th Street
Little Rock, AR 72201 USA
Contact: Sarah Tackett, Owner
T 1 501 374 6447
F 1 501 374 8903
W www.theagency-inc.com
E sarahtac@swbell.com

EXCEL MODELS AND TALENT
8201 Cantrell Road, Suite 215
Little Rock, AR 72227 USA
Contact: Melissa Moody
T 1 501 227 4232
F 1 501 228 5084
E excellr@cs.com

FERGUSON MODELING & TALENT AGENCY
1100 West 34th Street
Little Rock, AR 72206 USA
Contact: Erma Ferguson
T 1 501 375 3519
F 1 501 375 1132

THE MODEL CENTER
715 Sherman, Suite 13
Little Rock, AR 72202 USA
Contact: Scie Ward
T 1 501 372 6711
F 1 501 372 6711
E scieward@msn.com

TERRY LONG MODELS
P.O. Box 7353
Little Rock, AR 72217 USA
Contact: Terry Long Bogle
T 1 501 221 2202
F 1 501 224 4549
E TLmodels@aol.com

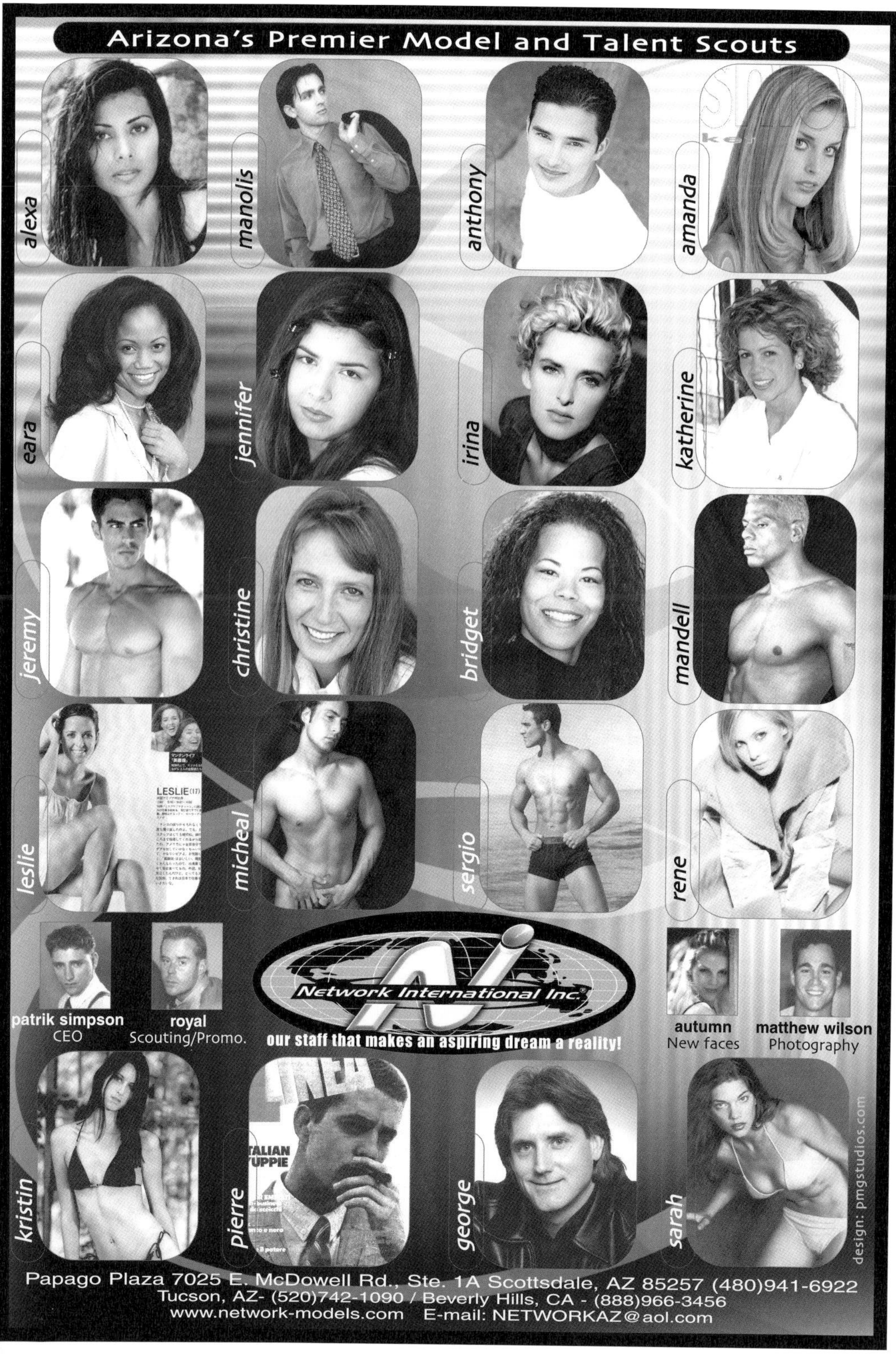
Arizona's Premier Model and Talent Scouts
alexa
manolis
anthony
amanda
eara
jennifer
irina
katherine
jeremy
christine
bridget
mandell
leslie
LESLIE(17)
micheal
sergio
rene
patrik simpson
CEO
royal
Scouting/Promo.
Network International Inc.
our staff that makes an aspiring dream a reality!
autumn
New faces
matthew wilson
Photography
kristin
pierre
ITALIAN YUPPIE
george
sarah
design: pmgstudios.com
Papago Plaza 7025 E. McDowell Rd., Ste. 1A Scottsdale, AZ 85257 (480)941-6922
Tucson, AZ- (520)742-1090 / Beverly Hills, CA - (888)966-3456
www.network-models.com E-mail: NETWORKAZ@aol.com

MODEL & TALENT AGENCIES

CALIFORNIA

John Robert Powers
30125 Agoura Road, Suite G
Agoura Hills, CA 91301 USA
T 1 818 735 8620
F 1 818 735 5759

EXTRAORDINAIRE MODELS & TALENT
200 New Stine Road, Suite 200
Bakersfield, CA 93309 USA
Contact: Voloney White
T 1 661 397 4440
F 1 661 397 1157
W www.exmodeltalent.com
E vawhite@exmodeltalent.com

MCCRIGHT TALENT AGENCY
1011 Stine Road
Bakersfield, CA 93309 USA
Contact: Ann McCright, Agent
T 1 661 835 1305
F 1 661 835 1329

JAB MODELS
5038 N Parkway Calabases, Suite 501
Calabasas, CA 91302 USA
Contact: Karen Monaco
T 1 818 876 0804
F 1 818 876 0803
W www.jabmodels.com
E karen@jabmodels.com

The Beverly Agency
371 Mobile Avenue
Camarillo, CA 93010 USA
T 1 805 445 9262
F 1 805 987 3469

ELEGANCE TALENT AGENCY & MODEL MANAGEMENT
2763 State Street
Carlsbad, CA 92008 USA
Contact: Pam Pahnke
SAG/AFTRA Franchised
T 1 760 434 3397
F 1 760 434 1406

PULSE MANAGEMENT
300 Carlsbad Village Drive, Suite 108-A31
Carlsbad, CA 92008-2999 USA
Contact: Stacey Eastman or Shayna Edwards
T 1 888 727 6569 US
T 1 760 521 4193 INTL
F 1 760 754 1269
W www.pulsemanagement.com
E info@pulsemanagement.com

John Robert Powers
20 Independence Circle
Chico, CA 95973 USA
T 1 530 879 5900
F 1 530 879 5905

Max Model & Talent Management
980 Springfield Street
Costa Mesa, CA 92626 USA
T 1 714 641 7430
F 1 714 641 7430

THE MORGAN AGENCY
129 West Wilson Street, Suite 202
Costa Mesa, CA 92627 USA
Contact: Keith Lewis
T 1 949 574 1100
F 1 949 574 1122
E morgan@themorganagency.com
***See Ad This Section.**

MARI SMITH PRESENTS, INC
MODEL & TALENT AGENCY
101 State Place, Suite D
Escondido, CA 92029 USA
Contact: Sandi Smith
T 1 760 745 1627
T 1 888 506 6060 Clients Only
F 1 760 432 8746
W www.nationwidemodels.com
E sandi@nationwidemodels.com
***See Ad Under San Diego Area.**

BARBIZON OF FRESNO
4844 N 1st Street, Suite 104
Fresno CA 93726 USA
Contact: Steven Neubauer, Owner
T 1 559 225 4883
F 1 559 225 4867
W www.modelingschools.com/fresno
E sneub90766@aol.com

Scream Entertainment Management
15500 Rockfield Boulevard
Irvine, CA 92618 USA
T 1 949 837 9900
F 1 949 837 5863

SMT MANAGEMENT/SELECT MODEL & TALENT
4000 Barranca Parkway, Suite 250
Irvine, CA 92604 USA
Contact: Petrina Milburn, Teens/Adults
Lisa Burdick, Kids
T 1 949 262 3293
T 1 949 262 3422
F 1 949 262 3294
W www.smtmanagement.com
E select@smtmanagement.com

John Robert Powers
24310 Moulton Parkway, Suite i
Laguna Hills, CA 92653 USA
T 1 949 609 1600
F 1 949 609 1601

JET SET MANAGEMENT GROUP INC
2160 Avenida De La Playa
La Jolla, CA 92037 USA
Contact: Cindy Kauanui
T 1 858 551 9393
F 1 858 551 9392
W www.jet-set.com
E cindy@jet-set.com

Nouveau Model Management
909 Prospect Street, Suite 239
La Jolla, CA 92037 USA
T 1 619 456 1400
F 1 619 456 1969

CHIC MODELS
5353 Paoli Way
Long Beach, CA 90803 USA
Contact: Patty Mezin
T 1 562 433 8097
F 1 562 433 2224
W www.chicmodels.com
E faces@chicmodels.com

Barbizon
4050 Katella Avuenue, Suite 213
Los Alamitos, CA 90720 USA
T 1 714 625 3540
F 1 562 799 9405

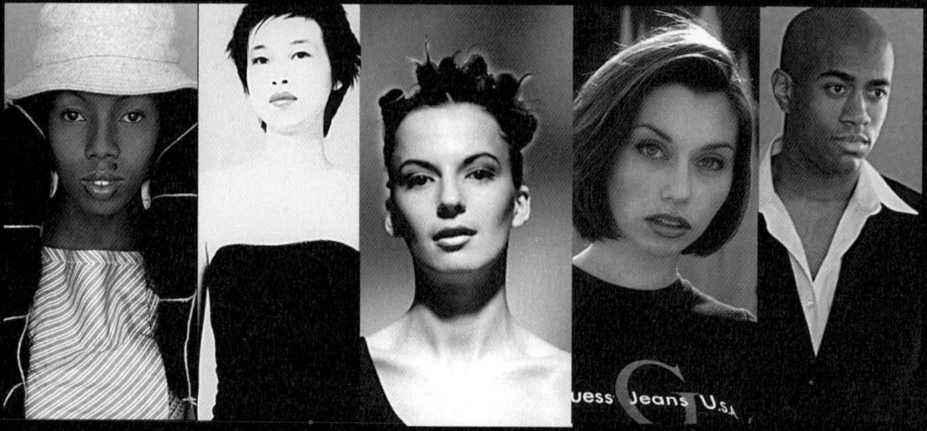

MODELING AGENCIES

LOS ANGELES AREA

MODEL AND TALENT AGENCY

AFFINITY

SAN FRANCISCO • LOS ANGELES • NEW YORK • CHICAGO

AFFINITY MODEL & TALENT
8721 Santa Monica Boulevard, Suite 27,
West Hollywood, CA 90069-4511 USA
Contact: Ross Kenneth
High Fashion/Print Specialists, Film and Television Specialists. Both Local and National, TA# 3562
TF 1 888 252 7000 Toll Free
F 1 310 388 5444
W www.affinitytalent.com
W www.affinitymodels.com
E info@affinitytalent.com
***See Ad This Section.**

AGENCY 2000
1150 South Spaulding Avenue, 2nd Floor
Los Angeles, CA 90019 USA
Contact: Kurt Clements
T 1 323 634 0475
F 1 323 634 0519
E AMODEL2000@aol.com
***See Ad This Section.**

BASS INTERNATIONAL MODELSCOUT
10877 Palms Blvd, Suite 1
Los Angeles, CA 90034 USA
Contact: Sandi Bass
Representing: Agence Presse, Tokyo
T 1 310 839 1097
F 1 310 839 1097
E sandibass@earthlink.net

BBA MODELS • A DIVISION OF BOBBY BALL AGENCY
4342 Lankershim Boulevard
Universal City, CA 91602 USA
Print: Christine Tarallo/Joy Hadjian
Commercials: Patty Grana-Miller
T 1 818 506 8188
F 1 818 506 8588
W www.bbamodels.com
E bbamodels@castnet.com

Bleu Model Management
8564 Wilshire Boulevard
Beverly Hills, CA 90211 USA
T 1 310 854 0088
F 1 310 854 0033

LOS ANGELES MODELING AGENCIES

C' LA VIE MODELS
7507 Sunset Boulevard, Suite 201
Los Angeles, CA 90046 USA
Contact: Steve Landry
T 1 323 969 0541
F 1 323 969 0401
E slandry@castnet.com

CASTOR MODEL & TALENT MANAGEMENT
468 N Camden Drive, Suite 200
Beverly Hills, CA 90210 USA
Contact: Carlos Moran
T 1 310 285 5361
F 1 310 388 1223
E carlos@castorentertainment.com

CHAMPAGNE / TROTT MODEL MANAGEMENT
9250 Wilshire Boulevard, Suite 303
Beverly Hills, CA 90210 USA
Contact: Francine Champagne or Valerie Trott
T 1 310 275 0067
F 1 310 275 3131
W www.champagnetrott.com
E models@champagnetrott.com
***See Ad This Section.**

CLICK MODELS OF LOS ANGELES
9057 Nemo Street
West Hollywood CA 90069 USA
T 1 310 246 0800
F 1 310 858 1357
E glenn@clickmodelsla.com

Colleen Cler Modeling Agency
120 S Victory Boulevard, Suite 206
Burbank, CA 91502 USA
T 1 818 841 7943
F 1 818 841 4541

Colours Model & Talent Agency
8344 1/2 West 3rd Street
Los Angeles, CA 90048 USA
T 1 323 658 7072
F 1 323 658 7074

Crew Men Agency
8344 1/2 West 3rd Street
Los Angeles, CA 90048
T 323 658 7280
F 323 658 7074

>>

CUNNINGHAM, ESCOTT & DIPENE
10635 Santa Monica Blvd, Suite 135
Los Angeles, CA 90025 USA
Contact: Carol Scott, Print Division
T 1 310 475 7573
F 1 310 475 6146
W www.cedtalent.com
E info@cedtalent.com

ELITE MODEL MANAGEMENT
345 North Maple Drive, Suite 397
Beverly Hills, CA 90210 USA
T 1 310 274 9395
F 1 310 278 7520
W www.elitelosangeles.com
E elitemodels@elitelosangeles.com

EMPIRE MODEL MANAGEMENT
1875 Century Park East, Suite 2250
Los Angeles, CA 90067 USA
T 1 310 843 5234
F 1 310 843 0123

EQUINOX MODELS
8961 Sunset Boulevard, PH
Los Angeles, CA 90069 USA
T 1 310 274 5088
F 1 310 274 5095
W www.equinoxmodels.com
E equinoxmodels@mindspring.com

FORD MODELS INC
8826 Burton Way
Beverly Hills, CA 90211 USA
T 1 310 276 8100
F 1 310 276 9299

GLAMOUR MODELS INC / GLAMOUR KIDS
211 South Beverly Drive, Suite 110
Beverly Hills, CA 90212 USA
Contact: Michael Douglas
Catalog & Commercial Print
T 1 310 859 3989
F 1 310 205 9188
W www.glamourmodelsinc.com

Howard Talent West
10657 Riverside Drive
Toluca Lake, CA 91602 USA
T 1 818 766 5300
F 1 818 760 3328

Jana Luker Agency
1923 1/2 Westwood Boulevard, Suite 3
Los Angeles, CA 90025-4613 USA
T 1 310 441 2822
F 1 310 441 2820

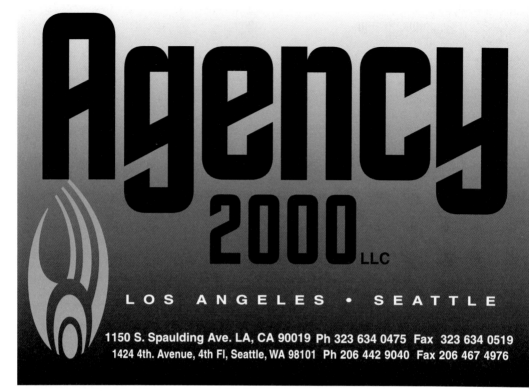

LOS ANGELES MODELING AGENCIES

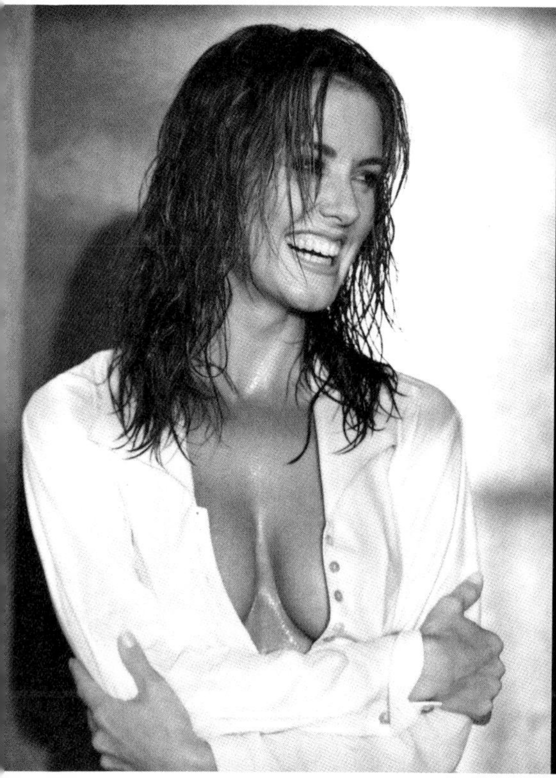

BRAND

model & talent agency, inc.

www.brandmodelandtalent.com

Full Service Talent Agency • SAG Franchise

(714) 850-1158 Phone
(714) 850-0806 Fax

1520 Brookhollow Drive Suite 39
Santa Ana California 92705

Linda....Print • Phyllis....Classics
Lisa....Plus Size • Marlyn....New Faces
Holly....Kids • Jennifer....Commercial & V/O
Dana....Tradeshow • Kelly....Runway &
Promotions • Jo....Accounting

Patty & Craig Brand...Proudly Serving
Clients Nationwide Since 1986

JET SET MANAGEMENT GROUP INC • LOS ANGELES
9255 Sunset Boulevard, Suite 727
W Hollywood, CA 90069
Contact: Bob Dixon, Director
T 1 310 786 7877
F 1 310 786 7872

John Robert Powers
9220 Sunset Boulevard, Suite 100
W Hollywood, CA 90069 USA
T 1 310 858 3300
F 1 310 858 3310

JVP MODEL & TALENT MANAGEMENT
171 N Labrea
Los Angeles, CA 90301 USA
T 1 310 330 9373
F 1 310 330 9375
W www.jvpmanagement.com
E jvpmngmt@pacbell.net

CHAMPAGNE (TROTT

9250 Wilshire Blvd, Suite 303
Beverly Hills, California 90212
310.275.0067 (T)
310.275.3131 (F)
models@champagnetrott.com (E)

L.A. MANAGEMENT
7700 Sunset Boulevard
Los Angeles, CA 90046 USA
T 1 323 436 7711
F 1 323 436 7755
W www.lamodels.com
E management@lamodels.com

L.A. MODELS
7700 Sunset Boulevard
Los Angeles, CA 90046 USA
Contact: Heinz Holba
T 1 323 436 7700
F 1 323 436 7755
W www.lamodels.com
E management@lamodels.com
***See Ad This Section.**

MATCH MODELS
7204 1/2 Melrose Avenue, Suite C
Los Angeles, CA 90046 USA
Contact: Tracey
T 1 323 525 3035
F 1 323 525 3040

Meridian Models & Talent Agency
215 S LaCienega Boulevard, PH
Beverly Hills, CA 90211 USA
T 1 310 289 8011
F 1 310 289 8136

MMI
1219 Morningside Drive
Manhattan Beach, CA 90266 USA
T 1 310 901 7096
F 1 310 362 8921
W www.modelmgmt.com
E mmi@modelmgmt.com

Model Team Agency
12435 Oxnard Street
N Hollywood, CA 91606 USA
T 1 818 755 0026
F 1 818 755 0027

MODELS LOS ANGELES
270 N Canon Drive, Suite 1267
Beverly Hills, CA 90210 USA
T 1 310 680 1713
F 1 310 680 1710

Models Guild of CA
8489 West 3rd Street, Suite 1035
Los Angeles, CA 90048 USA
T 1 323 801 2132
F 1 323 801 2133

>>

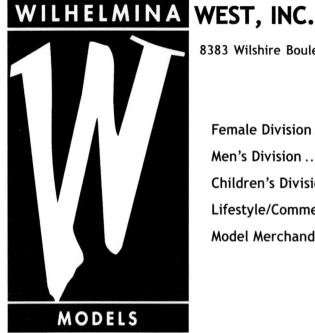

THE MORGAN AGENCY
129 West Wilson Street, Suite 202
Costa Mesa, CA 92627 USA
Contact: Keith Lewis
T 1 949 574 1100
F 1 949 574 1122
E morgan@themorganagency.com
*See Ad This Section.

NETWORK INTERNATIONAL INC
319 S Robertson
Beverly Hills, CA 90211 USA
Contact: Patrik Simpson / Peter Castillo / Royal Robins
T 1 888 966 3456
F 1 818 889 5242
W www.network-models.com
E NETWORKAZ@aol.com
*See Ad This Section.

NEXT MANAGEMENT • BEVERLY HILLS
8447 Wilshire Boulevard, Suite 301
Beverly Hills, CA 90211 USA
T 1 323 782 0010
T: 1 323 782 0021 Artist LA
F 1 323 782 0035
W www.nextmodelmanagement.com
*See Ad This Section.

NOUS MODEL MANAGEMENT
117 North Robertson Boulevard
Los Angeles, CA 90048 USA
Contact: Katy Strouk / Kenya Knight
T 1 310 385 6900
F 1 310 385 6910
W www.nous.net
E katy@nous.net
E kenya@nous.net

Odyssey model management

ODYSSEY MODELS
2050 S Bundy Drive, Suite 200B,
W Los Angeles, CA 90025 USA
Contact: Sara Gaynor
T 1 310 882 0706
F 1 310 820 1055
W www.odysseymodels.com
E info@odysseymodels.com

Otto Model Management
1460 N Sweetzer
Los Angeles, CA 90069 USA
T 1 323 650 2200
F 1 323 650 1134

Playboy Models
9242 Beverly Boulevard
Beverly Hills, CA 91210 USA
T 1 310 246 4000
F 1 310 246 4050

Q MODEL MANAGEMENT
6100 Wilshire Boulevard
Los Angeles, CA 90048 USA
T 1 323 468 2255
F 1 323 468 2540
W www.qmodels.com
E la@qmodels.com

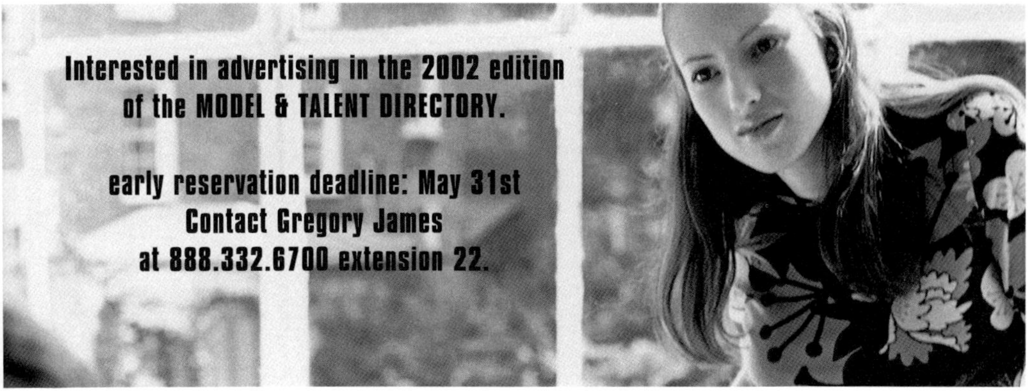
Interested in advertising in the 2002 edition
of the MODEL & TALENT DIRECTORY.
early reservation deadline: May 31st
Contact Gregory James
at 888.332.6700 extension 22.

VE MODELS AGENCY
9615 Brighton Way, Suite 302
Beverly Hills, CA 90210 USA
Contact: Vivian Damo
T 1 310 247 4500
F 1 310 247 4505
W www.vemodels.com
E vemodels@aol.com

VISAGE • LOS ANGELES
28957 Crest Ridge Road
R.P.V., CA 90275 USA
Contact: Mariko Tatsumi
T 1 310 377 8039
F 1 310 377 6613
E visage@bigplanet.com

WARNING MODEL MANAGEMENT
9009 Beverly Boulevard, Suite 103
Los Angeles, CA 90048 USA
Contact: Steve Chamberlin
T 1 310 860 9969
F 1 310 860 9978
E WarningLA@aol.com

WILHELMINA WEST INC
8383 Wilshire Boulevard
Beverly Hills, CA 90211 USA
T 1 323 655 0909 Women/Print
T 1 323 655 6508 Men/Print
T 1 212 477 3112 Kids Search Contest
T 1 212 477 3112 Teen Search Contest
T 1 800 889 6633 Model Merchandise
F 1 323 653 2255
***See Ad This Section.**

PERSONAL MANAGERS

CALIFORNIA

Chancellor Entertainment
10600 Holman Avenue, Suite 1
Los Angeles, CA 90024 USA
T 1 310 474 4521
F 1 310 470 9273

Dakota Management Group
269 S Beverly Drive, Suite 904
Beverly Hills, CA 90212 USA
T 1 714 777 6577

JDS Talent Management
15901 Condor Ridge Road
Santa Clarita, CA 91351 USA
T 1 661 298 4050
F 1 661 298 8655

MCD L.A. MANAGEMENT
11661 San Vicente Boulevard, Suite 609
Los Angeles, CA 90049 USA
T 1 310 454 3300
F 1 310 454 1954
E creativeservices@matthau.com

Scappatori Management
48 Via La Cumbre
Greenbrae, CA 94904-1331 USA
T 1 800 451 5813
F 1 800 236 7071

TALENT AGENCIES

CALIFORNIA

Abrams Artists Agency
9200 Sunset Boulevard, 11th Floor
Los Angeles, CA 90069 USA
T 1 310 859 0625
F 1 310 276 6193

Agency For Performing Arts
9000 Sunset Boulevard, Suite 1200
Los Angeles, CA 90069 USA
T 1 310 888 4200
F 1 310 888 4242

Aimee Entertainment
15000 Ventura Boulevard, Suite 340
Sherman Oaks, CA 91403 USA
T 1 818 783 9115

Alese Marshall Agency
22730 Hawthorne Boulevard, Suite 201
Torrance, CA 90505 USA
T 1 310 378 1223

Amsel Eisenstadt & Frazier
5757 Wilshire Boulevard, Suite 510
Los Angeles, CA 90036 USA
T 1 323 939 1188
F 1 323 939 0630

Ann Waugh Talent Agency
4741 Laurel Canyon Boulevard, Suite 200
N Hollywood, CA 91607 USA
T 1 818 980 0141

Arlene Thornton & Associates
12001 Ventura Place, Suite 201
Studio City, CA 91604 USA
T 1 818 760 6688

Artists Agency
10000 Santa Monica Boulevard, Suite 305
Los Angeles, CA 90067 USA
T 1 310 277 7779
F 1 310 785 9338

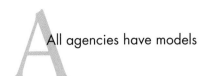

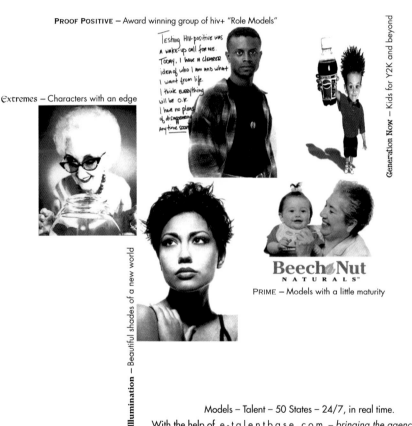

Artists Group
10100 Santa Monica Boulevard, Suite 2490
Los Angeles, CA 90067 USA
T 1 310 552 1100

Artists Management West
1800 East Garry Street, Suite 101
Santa Ana, CA 92705 USA
T 1 949 261 7557

A Total Acting Experience
20501 Ventura Boulevard, Suite 399
Woodland Hills, CA 91364 USA
T 1 818 340 9249

Berzon Talent
336 E 17th Street
Costa Mesa, CA 92627 USA
T 1 949 631 5936

Beverly Hecht Agency
12001 Ventura Place, Suite 320
Studio City, CA 91604 USA
T 1 818 505 1192
F 1 818 505 1590

Bobby Ball Talent Agency
4342 Lankershim Boulevard
Universal City, CA 91602 USA
T 1 818 506 8188
F 1 818 506 8588

Bresler Kelly & Associates
11500 W Olympic Boulevard, Suite 510
Los Angeles, CA 90064 USA
T 1 310 479 5611
F 1 310 479 3775

C' LA VIE TALENT
7507 Sunset Boulevard, Suite 201
Los Angeles, CA 90046 USA
Contact: Steve Landry
T 1 323 969 0541
F 1 323 969 0401
E slandry@castnet.com

Career Artists International
11030 Ventura Boulevard, Suite 3
Studio City, CA 91604 USA
T 1 818 980 1315

Castle Hill Enterprises
1101 S Orlando Avenue
Los Angeles, CA 90035 USA
T 1 323 653 3535

Cavaleri & Associates
405 Riverside DRive, Suite 200
Burbank, CA 91506 USA
T 1 818 955 9300

CHAMPAGNE/TROTT TALENT AGENCY
9250 Wilshire Boulevard, Suite 303
Beverly Hills, CA 90210 USA
Contact: Kelly Gursey
T 1 310 205 3111
F 1 310 205 3431
W www.champagnetrott.com
E models@champagnetrott.com

Chasin Agency
8899 Beverly Boulevard, Suite 716
Los Angeles, CA 90048 USA
T 1 310 278 7505
F 1 310 275 6685

CNA & Associates
1925 Century Park East, Suite 750
Los Angeles, CA 90067 USA
T 1 310 556 4343
F 1 310 556 4633

Coast to Coast Talent Group
3350 Barham Boulevard
Los Angeles, CA 90068 USA
T 1 323 845 9200

Coppage Company
3500 W Olive Avenue, Suite 1420
Burbank, CA 91505 USA
T 1 818 953 4163

Coralie Jr Agency
4789 Vineland Avenue, Suite 100
N Hollywood, CA 91602 USA
T 1 818 766 9501

THE COSDEN AGENCY
3518 Cahuenga Boulevard West, Suite 200
Los Angeles, CA 90068 USA
Contact: John McCormick
T 1 323 874 7200
F 1 323 874 7800
E jmccormick@cosdenagency.com

Creative Artists Agency
9830 Wilshire Boulevard
Beverly Hills, CA 90212 USA
T 1 310 288 4545

CUNNINGHAM, ESCOTT & DIPENE
10635 Santa Monica Blvd, Suite 130
Los Angeles, CA 90025 USA
Voice Over: Paul Doherty
On Camera: Linda Jenkins or Adrienne Berg
Children: Bob Preston
T 1 310 475 2111
T 1 310 475 3336 Children
F 1 310 475 1929
W www.cedtalent.com
E info@cedtalent.com

Dade/Schultz Associates
12302 Sarah Street, Suite 19
Studio City, CA 91604 USA
T 1 818 760 3100
F 1 818 760 1395

Dale Garrick International
8831 Sunset Boulevard, Suite 402
Los Angeles, CA 90069 USA
T 1 310 657 2661
F 1 310 657 3509

H. David Moss & Associates
733 N Seward Street, PH
Hollywood, CA 90038 USA
T 1 323 465 1234
F 1 323 465 1241

David Shapira & Associates
15301 Ventura Boulevard, Suite 345
Sherman Oaks, CA 91403 USA
T 1 818 906 0322
F 1 818 783 2562

Don Buchwald & Associates
6500 Wilshire Boulevard, Suite 2200
Los Angeles, CA 90048 USA
T 1 323 655 7400

Edwards & Associates
5455 Wilshire Boulevard, Suite 1614
Los Angeles, CA 90036 USA
T 1 323 964 0000
F 1 323 964 0210

EWCR & Associates
280 S Beverly Drive, Suite 400
Beverly Hills, CA 90212 USA
T 1 310 278 7222
F 1 310 278 4640

Film Artists Associates
13563 Ventura Boulevard, 2nd Floor
Sherman Oaks, CA 91423 USA
T 1 818 386 9669
F 1 818 386 9363

Flick East-West Talents Inc
9057 Nemo Street, Suite A
Los Angeles, CA 90069 USA
T 1 310 271 9111
F 1 310 858 1357

Gage Group
9255 Sunset Boulevard, Suite 515
Los Angeles, CA 90069 USA
T 1 310 859 8777
F 1 310 859 8166

Geddes Agency
8430 Santa Monica Boulevard, Suite 200
W Hollywood, CA 90069 USA
T 1 323 848 2700

George Jay Agency
6269 Selma Avenue, Suite 15
Los Angeles, CA 90028 USA
T 1 323 446 6665
F 1 323 462 6197

The Gerler Agency
3349 Cahuenga Boulevard W, Suite 1
Los Angeles, CA 90068 USA
T 1 323 850 7386
F 1 323 850 7490

Gersh Agency Inc
232 N Canon Drive
Beverly Hills, CA 90210 USA
T 1 310 274 6611
F 1 310 274 3923

Gold-Marshak-Liedtke
3500 W Olive Avenue, Suite 1400
Burbank, CA 91505 USA
T 1 818 972 4300

Gordon Rael Agency
9229 Sunset Boulevard
Los Angeles, CA 90069 USA
T 1 310 285 0572
F 1 310 285 0259

HWA Talent Representatives
1964 Westwood Boulevard, Suite 400
Los Angeles, CA 90025 USA
T 1 310 446 1313
F 1 310 446 1364

Henderson/Hogan Agency
247 S Beverly Drive, Suite 102
Beverly Hills, CA 90210 USA
T 1 310 274 7815
F 1 310 274 0751

Herb Tannen Associates
8370 Wilshire Boulevard, Suite 209
Beverly Hills, CA 90211 USA
T 1 323 782 0515
F 1 323 782 0811

IDENTITY TALENT AGENCY
2050 S Bundy Drive, Suite 200B
W Los Angeles, CA 90025 USA
Contact: Erik DeSando
T 1 310 882 6070
F 1 310 820 1055

>>

Innovative Artists
1505 10th Street
Santa Monica, CA 90401 USA
T 1 310 553 5200
F 1 310 557 2211

International Creative Management
8942 Wilshire Boulevard
Beverly Hills, CA 90211 USA
T 1 310 550 4000
F 1 310 550 4108

Iris Burton Agency
P.O. Box 15306
Beverly Hills, CA 90209 USA
T 1 310 288 0121

Irv Schecter Company
9300 Wilshire Boulevard, Suite 400
Beverly Hills, CA 90212 USA
T 1 310 278 8070
F 1 310 278 1192

Jack Scagnetti Talent Agency
5118 Vineland Avenue, Suite 102
N Hollywood, CA 91601 USA
T 1 818 762 3871
F 1 818 761 6629

Page Management
P.O. Box 573040
Woodland Hills, CA 91357 USA
T 1 818 703 7328
F 1 818 883 4344

Judy Schoen Associates
606 N Larchmont Avenue, Suite 309
Los Angeles, CA 90004 USA
T 1 323 962 1950
F 1 323 461 8365

Ken Lindner & Associates
2049 Century Park E, Suite 3050
Los Angeles, CA 90067 USA
T 1 310 277 6023
F 1 310 277 5806

L.A. TALENT
7700 Sunset Boulevard
Los Angeles, CA 90046 USA
Contact: Heinz Holba
T 1 323 436 7777 TV
T 1 323 436 7778 Adult
T 1 323 436 7779 Kids
F 1 323 436 7700
W www.latalent.com
E adultcom@latalent.com

The Levin Agency
8484 Wilshire Boulevard, Suite 745
Beverly Hills, CA 90211 USA
T 1 323 653 7073
F 1 323 653 0280

Lovell & Associates
7095 Hollywood Boulevard, Suite 1006
Los Angeles, CA 90028-8903 USA
T 1 323 876 1560
F 1 323 876 1474

Media Artists Group
6404 Wilshire Boulevard, Suite 950
Beverly Hills, CA 90048 USA
T 1 323 658 5050
F 1 323 658 7871

Metropolitan Talent Agency
4526 Wilshire Boulevard
Los Angeles, CA 90010 USA
T 1 323 857 4500
F 1 323 857 4599

THE MORGAN AGENCY
129 West Wilson Street, Suite 202
Costa Mesa, CA 92627 USA
Contact: Keith Lewis
T 1 949 574 1100
F 1 949 574 1122
E morgan@themorganagency.com
***See Ad This Section.**

Omnipop Inc
10700 Ventura Boulevard, 2nd Floor
Studio City, CA 91604 USA
T 1 818 980 9267
F 1 818 980 9371

Osbrink Talent Agency
4343 Lankershim Boulevard, Suite 100
Universal City, CA 91602 USA
T 1 818 760 2488
F 1 818 760 0991

Paradigm
10100 Santa Monica Boulevard, 25th Floor
Los Angeles, CA 90067 USA
T 1 310 277 4400
F 1 310 277 7820

Paul Kohner Inc
9300 Wilshire Boulevard, Suite 555
Beverly Hills, CA 90212 USA
T 1 310 550 1060
F 1 310 276 1083

Privilege Talent Agency
9229 Sunset Boulevard, Suite 201
Los Angeles, CA 90069 USA
T 1 310 858 5277
F 1 310 858 5267

Progressive Artists Agency
400 S Beverly Drive, Suite 216
Beverly Hills, CA 90212 USA
T 1 310 553 8561
F 1 310 553 4726

Robert Light Agency
6404 Wilshire Boulevard, Suite 900
Los Angeles, CA 90048 USA
T 1 323 651 1777
F 1 323 651 4933

Sanders Agency Ltd
8831 Sunset Boulevard, Suite 304
Los Angeles, CA 90069-2109 USA
T 1 310 652 1119

Sandie Schnarr Talent
8500 Melrose Avenue, Suite 212
W Hollywood, CA 90069 USA
T 1 310 360 7680
F 1 310 360 7681

Sara Bennett Agency
6404 Hollywood Boulevard, Suite 316
Los Angeles, CA 90028 USA
T 1 323 965 9666

Savage Agency
6212 Banner Avenue
Hollywood, CA 90038 USA
T 1 323 461 8316
F 1 323 461 2417

Scappatori Management
5515 York Boulevard
Los Angeles, CA 90042-2403 USA
T 1 800 451 5813
F 1 800 236 7071

Schiowitz/Clay/Rose Inc
1680 Vine Street, Suite 614
Los Angeles, CA 90028 USA
T 1 323 463 7300
F 1 323 463 7355

Screen Artist Agency
12435 Oxnard Street
N Hollywood, CA 91606 USA
T 1 818 755 0026
F 1 818 755 0027

Screen Children's Agency
4000 W Riverside Drive, Suite A
Burbank, CA 91505 USA
T 1 818 846 4300
F 1 818 846 3745

Shapiro-Lichtman Inc
8827 Beverly Boulevard
Los Angeles, CA 90048 USA
T 1 310 859 8877
F 1 310 859 7153

Shirley Wilson & Associates
5410 Wilshire Boulevard, Suite 806
Los Angeles, CA 90036 USA
T 1 323 857 6977
F 1 323 857 6980

Silver Massetti & Szatmary/West
8730 Sunset Boulevard, Suite 440
Los Angeles, CA 90069 USA
T 1 310 289 0909
F 1 310 289 0990

Special Artists Agency
345 N Maple Drive, Suite 302
Beverly Hills, CA 90210 USA
T 1 310 859 9688

Stacey Lane Talent Agency
13455 Ventura Boulevard, Suite 240
Sherman Oaks, CA 91423 USA
T 1 818 501 2668

Starwil Talent
433 North Camden Drive, 4th Floor
Beverly Hills, CA 90210 USA
T 1 323 874 1239
F 1 323 874 1822

Stone/Manners Agency
8436 W 3rd Street, Suite 740
Los Angeles, CA 90048 USA
T 1 323 655 1313
F 1 323 655 7676

Sutton, Barth & Vennari
145 S Fairfax Avenue, Suite 310
Los Angeles, CA 90036 USA
T 1 323 938 6000
F 1 323 935 8671

Talent Group Inc
6300 Wilshire Boulevard, Suite 900
Los Angeles, CA 90048 USA
T 1 323 852 9559
F 1 323 852 9579

>>

Terry Lichtman Co
12216 Moorpark Street
Studio City, CA 91604 USA
T 1 818 655 9898
F 1 818 658 9899

Tisherman Agency Inc
6767 Forest Lawn Drive, Suite 101
Los Angeles, CA 90068 USA
T 1 323 850 6767
F 1 323 850 7340

Twentieth Century Artists
4605 Lankershim Boulevard, Suite 305
N Hollywood, CA 91602 USA
T 1 818 980 5118
F 1 818 980 5449

Tyler Kjar Agency
5116 Lankershim Boulevard
N Hollywood, CA 91601 USA
T 1 818 760 0321
F 1 818 760 0642

United Talent
9560 Wilshire Boulevard, Suite 500
Beverly Hills, CA 90212 USA
T 1 310 273 6700
F 1 310 247 1111

Vaughn D Hart & Associates
8899 Beverly Boulevard, Suite 815
Los Angeles, CA 90048 USA
T 1 310 273 7887
F 1 310 273 7924

William Carroll Agency
139 N South Fernando Boulevard, Suite A
Burbank, CA 91502 USA
T 1 818 845 3791
F 1 818 845 1769

William Kerwin Agency
1605 N Cahuenga Boulevard, Suite 202
Los Angeles, CA 90028 USA
T 1 323 469 5155
F 1 323 469 5907

William Morris Agency
151 El Camino Drive
Beverly Hills, CA 90212 USA
T 1 310 859 4000
F 1 310 859 4462

World Class Sports
880 Apollo Street, Suite 337
El Segundo, CA 90245 USA
T 1 310 535 9120
F 1 310 535 9128

W Randolph Clark Agency
13415 Ventura Boulevard, Suite 3
Sherman Oaks, CA 91423-3937 USA
T 1 818 385 0583
F 1 181 358 0599

Writers & Artists
8383 Wilshire Boulevard, Suite 550
Beverly Hills, CA 90211 USA
T 1 323 866 0900
F 1 323 866 1899

MODEL & TALENT AGENCIES

CALIFORNIA CONTINUED

Select Models
24022 Tobaro
Murrieta, CA 82562 USA
T 1 909 677 3992

PUBLIC MODELS
20101 SW Birch, Suite 130G
Newport Beach, CA 92660 USA
Contact: Daniel Jackson, Owner
T 1 949 250 4944
F 1 949 250 4958
E modelpub@aol.com

John Robert Powers
300 Esplanade Drive, Suite 1640
Oxnard, CA 93030 USA
T 1 805 983 1076
F 1 805 983 0738

Cindy Romano Modeling & Talent Agency
P.O. Box 1951
Palm Springs, CA 92263 USA
T 1 760 323 3333
F 1 760 322 6666

Dorothy Shreve Model & Talent Center
2101 N Starr Road
Palm Springs, CA 92262 USA
T 1 760 327 5855
F 1 760 320 2782

IMM-INTERNATIONAL MODEL MANAGEMENT
235 E Colorado Blvd, PMB 244
Pasadena, CA 91101 USA
Contact: Gus Castaneda
T 1 626 918 3836
F 1 626 568 1789
E guscastanedaimm@earthlink.net

John Robert Powers
150 S Los Robles Avenue, Suite 900
Pasadena, CA 91101 USA
T 1 626 817 0900
F 1 626 817 0921

Cathy Steele Model & Talent Management
1610 Oakpark Boulevard, Suite 2
Pleasant Hill, CA 94523 USA
T 1 925 932 4226
F 1 925 946 4603

WOW MODEL & TALENT MANAGEMENT
1610 Oakpark Blvd, Suite 2
Pleasant Hill, CA 94523 USA
Contact: Cathy Steele or Andrew Steinmeyer
T 1 925 946 4622
F 1 925 946 4603

NE' VON MODEL MANAGEMENT
3595 University Avenue, Suite A
Riverside, CA 92501 USA
Contact: Vanessa Von / Cecelia Gonzalez
T 1 909 684 1237
F 1 909 684 1237
E ne'vonmodelmgmt@yahoo.com

Sacramento

Barbizon
701 Howe Avenue, Suite H50
Sacramento, CA 95825 USA
T 1 916 920 4200
F 1 916 920 5471

CAST IMAGES TALENT AGENCY
2530 J Street, Suite 330
Sacramento, CA 95816-4849 USA
Contact: Chandra Bourne
T 1 916 444 9655
F 1 916 444 2093
W www.castimages.com
E chandra@castimages.com

JOHN ROBERT POWERS
2929 K Street, 3rd Floor
Sacramento, CA 95816 USA
Contact: Deborah Adragna
T 1 916 341 7700
F 1 916 341 7744
W www.johnrobertpowers.net

Just For Kids
1111 Howe Avenue, Suite 600
Sacramento, CA 95825 USA
T 1 916 929 4386
F 1 916 568 2784

San Diego

Artist Management
835 Fifth Avenue, Suite 411
San Diego, CA 92101-6137 USA
T 1 619 233 6655
F 1 619 233 5332

Barbizon
591 Camino de la Reina, Suite 1150
San Diego, CA 92108 USA
T 1 619 296 6366
F 1 619 296 3720

John Robert Powers
8910 University Center Lane, Suite 120
San Diego, CA 92122 USA
T 1 858 824 0700
F 1 858 824 0705

SAN DIEGO MODEL MANAGEMENT
438 Camino Del Rio South, Suite 116
San Diego, CA 92108 USA
Large Print Divisions in Women, Men, Kids. Also Commercial Print, Runway & Talent. 16 years experience with East Coast, European, and Asian photo crews - Call for model packet! Providing new face modeling talent to all major markets including LA, NY, Europe, and Japan. SAG/AFTRA
T 1 619 296 1018
F 1 619 296 3422
W www.sdmodel.com
E sdmm@eciti.com
***See Ad This Section.**

≫

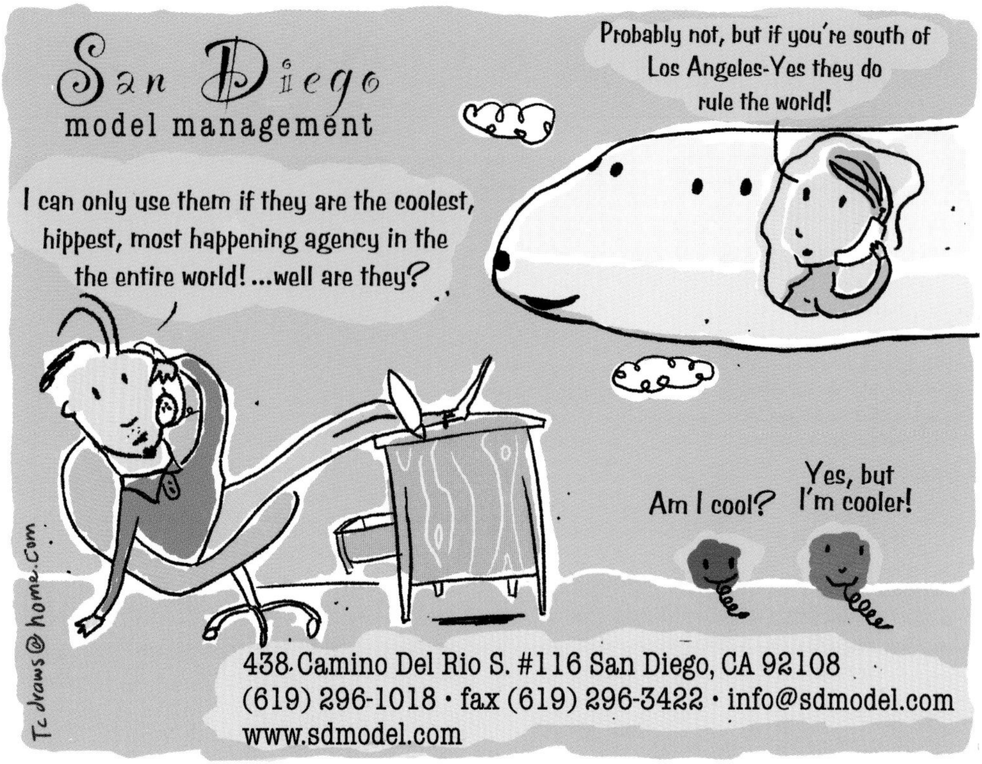

Shamon Freitas Model & Talent
9606 Tierra Grande, Suite 204
San Diego, CA 92126 USA
T 1 858 549 3955
F 1 858 549 7028

TINA REAL CASTING
3108 Fifth Avenue, Suite C
San Diego, CA 92103-5829 USA
Contact: Tina Real
Commercials • Film • Print
T 1 619 298 0544
F 1 619 298 0389
E tnreal@aol.com

San Francisco

MODEL AND TALENT AGENCY
AFFINITY
SAN FRANCISCO • LOS ANGELES • NEW YORK • CHICAGO

AFFINITY MODEL & TALENT
100 First Street, Suite 100-362
San Francisco, CA 94105 USA
Contact: Ross Kenneth
High Fashion/Print Specialists, Film and Television Specialists. Both Local and National, TA# 3562
TF 1 888 252 7000 Toll free
T 1 415 409 9991
F 1 415 449 3638
W www.affinitytalent.com
W www.affinitymodels.com
E info@affinitytalent.com
***See Ad This Section.**

BOOM! MODELS & TALENT AGENCY
2325 3rd Street, Suite 223
San Francisco, CA 94107 USA
Contact: Kristen E. Usich or John Hutcheson
SAG/AFTRA Franchised
T 1 415 626 6591
F 1 415 626 6594
W www.boomagency.com
E boommodels@aol.com

CITY MODEL MANAGEMENT INC
36 Clyde Street
San Francisco, CA 94107 USA
Contact: Sal A. Marquez Jr.
Mens: Ken Moore
Womens: Sheree Kirkeby
Kids/Talent: Evee Sosa
T 1 415 546 3160
T 1 415 536 0145 Accounting
T 1 323 461 5240 LA
F 1 415 546 3170
W www.citymodel.com
E city1@pacbell.net

INDUSTRY MODEL & TALENT MANAGEMENT
942 Market Street, Suite 506/507
San Francisco, CA 94102 USA
Contact: Eddie Cotillon / Russell Hong
T 1 415 986 6151
F 1 415 986 7335
E industrymodels@hotmail.com

John Robert Powers
26 O'Farrell Street, 6th Floor
San Francisco, CA 94108 USA
T 1 415 362 8260
F 1 415 248 3909

MITCHELL AGENCY INC
323 Geary Street, Suite 302
San Francisco, CA 94102 USA
Contact: Ms. Troy Solarek
T 1 415 395 9291
T 1 415 395 9475 TV Dept
F 1 415 395 9556

SAN FRANCISCO TOP MODELS & TALENT
870 Market Street, Suite 1076
San Francisco, CA 94102 USA
Contact: Belinda Irons
T 1 415 391 1800
F 1 415 391 2012
E sftoptalent@aol.com

STARS, THE AGENCY
23 Grant Avenue, 4th Floor
San Francisco, CA 94108 USA
Contact: Lynn, Kristin or Scott Claxon
T 1 415 421 6272
F 1 415 421 7620
W www.starsagency.com
E scottc@starsagency.com
E kristinc@starsagency.com

Tonry Talent
885 Bryant Street, Suite 201
San Francisco, CA 94103 USA
T 1 415 543 3797
F 1 415 957 9656

• • • • • • • • • • •

HALVORSON MODEL MANAGEMENT
2858 Stevens Creek Boulevard, Suite 209
San Jose, CA 95128 USA
Contact: Traci Halvorson
T 1 408 983 1038
F 1 408 983 0910
W www.hmmodels.com
E hmmodels@aol.com

John Robert Powers
1600 Saratoga Avenue
San Jose, CA 95129 USA
T 1 408 871 8709
F 1 408 871 9238

John Robert Powers
2410 San Ramon Valley Boulevard, Suite 110
San Ramon, CA 94583 USA
T 1 925 837 9000
F 1 925 743 4415

BRAND MODEL & TALENT AGENCY
1520 Brookhollow Drive, Suite 39
Santa Ana, CA 92705 USA
Contact: Patty Brand
T 1 714 850 1158
F 1 714 850 0806
*See Ad Under LA Modeling Agencies.

The Jacqueline Agency
2919 W Pendleton Avenue
Santa Ana, CA 92704 USA
T 1 714 751 2450
F 1 714 751 2492

Susan Lane Agency, Inc.
14071 Windsor Place
Santa Ana, CA 92705 USA
T 1 714 731 4560
F 1 714 731 5223

>>

CALIFORNIA

Santa Barbara Models & Talent
2026 Cliff Drive, Suite 226
Santa Barbara, CA 93109 USA
T 1 805 963 1625
F 1 805 965 0553

Santa Rosa

BELLISSIMA MODEL & TALENT MANAGEMENT
1055 West College Avenue, Suite 334
Santa Rosa, CA 95401 USA
Contact: Susan Berosh
T 1 707 523 0819
F 1 707 523 2490
W www.bellissima.com
E model@bellissima.com

John Robert Powers
416 B Street, Suite C
Santa Rosa, CA 95401 USA
T 1 707 571 2400
F 1 707 571 5980

JULIE NATION ACADEMY
MODEL & TALENT MANAGEMENT
2455 Bennett Valley Road, Suite 110A
Santa Rosa, CA 95404 USA
Contact: Julie Nation
T 1 707 575 8585
F 1 707 575 8596
W www.julienation.com
E jnation@sonic.net

Panda Talent Agency
3721 Hoen Avenue
Santa Rosa, CA 95405 USA
T 1 707 576 0711
F 1 707 544 2765

Patricia Rile Models & Talent
4716 Foulger Drive
Santa Rosa, CA 95405 USA
T 1 707 537 8247
F 1 707 539 9290

• • • • • • • • • •

Midwest Talent
11211 Cohasset Street
Sun Valley, CA 91352 USA
T 1 818 765 3785
F 1 818 765 2903

John Robert Powers
27200 Tourney Road, Suite 105
Valencia, CA 91355 USA
T 1 661 286 1360
F 1 661 286 1370

AMBIANCE MODELS & TALENT
440 North Mountain Avenue, Suite 201
Upland, CA 91786 USA
Contact: Marti Raymond
T 1 909 931 3939
F 1 909 931 7939
W www.ambiance-inc.com

MODEL & TALENT AGENCIES

COLORADO

MODELS • ASPEN
P.O. Box 1733
Aspen, CO 81612-1733 USA
Contact: Rob Cloos, President
T 1 970 544 3557
F 1 970 925 4191
W www.modelsaspen.com

Colorado Springs

John Robert Powers
14231 E 4th Avenue, Bldg 1, Suite 200
Aurora, CO 80011 USA
T 1 303 340 2838
F 1 303 340 2848

John Robert Powers
4905 N Union Boulevard, Suite 202
Colorado Springs, CO 80918 USA
T 1 719 268 6633
F 1 719 260 8034

The Agency Downtown Company
422 East Vermijo Street, Suite 401
Colorado Springs, CO 80903 USA
T 1 719 884 0401
F 1 719 884 0421

MTA
1026 W Colorado Avenue
Colorado Springs, CO 80904 USA
T 1 719 577 4704
F 1 719 520 1952

VISUAL MODEL & TALENT MANAGEMENT
3645 Jeannine Drive, Suite 221
Colorado Springs, CO 80917-8011
Contact: Pepper or Michael
T 1 719 572 9096
F 1 719 574 6661
W www.mlamtc.com

Denver

Barbizon
7535 E Hampden Avenue
Denver, CO 80231 USA
T 1 303 337 6952
F 1 303 337 7955

DONNA BALDWIN TALENT, INC.
2150 W 29th Avenue, Suite 200
Denver, CO 80211 USA
Contact: Donna Baldwin
T 1 303 561 1199
F 1 303 561 1337
W www.donnabaldwin.com
E info@donnabaldwin.com
***See Ad This Section.**

John Casablancas/MTM
7600 E Eastman Avenue, Suite 100
Denver, CO 80231 USA
T 1 303 337 5100

Kidskits Inc
136 Kalamath
Denver, CO 80223 USA
T 1 303 446 8200
F 1 303 446 2629

MAXIMUM • A TALENT AGENCY
1660 S Albion Street, Suite 1004
Denver, CO 80222 USA
Contact: Rob Lail / Paula Block
T 1 303 691 2344
F 1 303 691 2488
W www.maxtalent.com
E info@maxtalent.com

MIRAGE TALENT AGENCY
2509 South Clermont Street
Denver, CO 80222 USA
Contact: Kent Allen
T 1 303 504 4581
F 1 303 753 1952
W www.miragetalent.com
E miragetalent@aol.com

• • • • • • • • • •

Ascent Models & Talent
7887 E Bellevue Avenue, Suite 1100
Englewood, CO 80111 USA
T 1 303 228 1622
F 1 303 228 2281

Petrell Model Management
4195 South Inca Street
Englewood, CO 80110-4513 USA
T 1 800 451 5813
F 1 800 236 7071

MODEL & TALENT AGENCIES

CONNECTICUT

JOHN CASABLANCAS
1263 Wilbur Cross Highway
Berlin, CT 06037 USA
Contact: Tina Kiniry, President
T 1 860 828 7577
F 1 860 828 5927

COASTAL MODELS LTD
2012 King's Highway East
Fairfield, CT 06430 USA
Contact: Marty Kanawall
T 1 203 254 7722
T 1 203 334 6944
F 1 203 254 7722
W www.coastalmodels.com
E coastalmod@aol.com

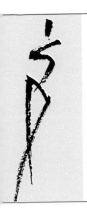

AMERICAN MALE MODEL & TALENT
61 Center Drive
Greenwich, CT 06870-1444 USA
Contact: Roger Jewell, Director
Representing & Scouting:
MODELS, ACTORS, BODYBUILDERS & ATHLETES
T 1 800 764 1020
F 1 877 625 3329
F 1 877 MALE FAX
E MALEMODELAGENT@AOL.COM

WSG Management
23 Thomes Street
Rowayton, CT 06853 USA
T 1 203 899 1718
F 1 203 227 6170

JOHNSTON AGENCY
50 Washington Street
S Norwalk, CT 06854 USA
Contact: Esther Johnston
T 1 203 838 6188
F 1 203 838 6642

BLUSH MODELS MANAGEMENT LLC
2 Pomperaug Office Park, Suite 102, Main Street S
Southbury, CT 06488 USA
Contact: Eli Shamsi, Director
Mailing: P.O. Box 1005, Southbury, CT 06488 USA
T 1 203 264 7782
T 1 203 267 7686 Clients Only
F 1 203 264 7782
W www.blushmodels.com
E agency_director@blushmodels.com

Actual Talent
1260 New Britain Avenue
West Hartford, CT 06110 USA
T 1 860 920 5322
F 1 860 561 2473

MCDONALD/RICHARDS • CONNECTICUT
5 River Road, Suite 317
Wilton, CT 06897 USA
Contact: Tracy Denard
Commercial Print/Catalog
T 1 203 377 7387
W www.mcdonaldrichards.com
*See Ad Under NYC Modeling Agencies Section.

VARIETY/CIRCUS AGENCIES

CONNECTICUT

GINAMARIE TALENT & ENTERTAINMENT
565 Kings Highway
Fairfield, CT 06430 USA
Contact: Jaya
T 1 800 737 0797
T 1 203 335 2121
F 1 203 335 3771
"You Name It...We've Got It!"

MODEL & TALENT AGENCIES

DELEWARE

Barbizon
17B Trolley Square
Wilmington, DE 19806 USA
T 1 302 658 6666
F 1 302 658 6658

START MODEL CONSULTANTS
1632 Savannah Road, Suite 12
Lewes, DE 19958 USA
Contact: George Brewer
T 1 302 644 3550
F 1 302 644 3575
W www.startmodels.com
E startmodels209@cs.com

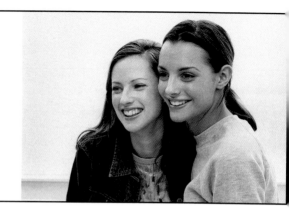

MODEL & TALENT AGENCIES

DISTRICT OF COLUMBIA

Actors & Models of Washington
906 D Street NE
Washington, DC 20002 USA
T 1 202 333 3560
F 1 202 544 2856

T.H.E. ARTIST AGENCY
3333 K Street NW, Suite 50
Washington, DC 20007 USA
Contact: Elizabeth McDavitt-Centenari
T 1 202 342 0933
F 1 202 342 6471
E info@theartistagency.com

MODEL & TALENT AGENCIES

FLORIDA

ARTHURARTHUR INC
6542 U.S. Highway 41 North, Suite 205A
Apollo Beach, FL 33572 USA
Contact: Jeremy Foster-Fell, CEO
or Diana Arthur, President
SAG Francised / FL Lic#: 617
T 1 813 645 9700
F 1 813 645 9797
E ArtArtInc@aol.com
***See Ad This Section.**

Studio On The Gulf
10421 Kentucky
Bonita Springs, FL 34135 USA
T 1 941 498 7386
F 1 941 498 1737

Barbizon
2240 Woolbright Road, Suite 300
Boynton Beach, FL 33426 USA
T 1 561 369 8600
F 1 561 369 1299

>>

IT'S TOTALLY YOU, INC
427 SE 16th Place, Suite 3
Cape Coral, FL 33904 USA
Contact: Claudia C. Hoh, Director
T 1 941 541 9111
F 1 941 772 5754
W www.itstotallyyou.com
E director@itstotallyyou.com

LATIN'S HISPANIC TALENT
3001 SW 28 Lane, Suite 1
Coconut Grove, FL 33133 USA
Contact: Carlos Segui, Director or Marisol Mata
T 1 305 567 9567
F 1 305 567 9727
W www.latinstalent.com
E carlos@latinstalent.com

Gabriel Productions International
2115 Le Juene Road
Coral Gables, FL 33134 USA
T 1 305 444 1999
F 1 305 444 9495

BOCA TALENT & MODEL AGENCY
829 SE 9th Street
Deerfield Beach, FL 33441 USA
Contact: Anita Spiegel
SAG • AFTRA • AEA, FL Lic#: TA0000038
T 1 954 428 4677
F 1 954 429 9203
E BCA100@aol.com

Ft Lauderdale

AVENUE PRODUCTIONS INC MODEL & TALENT AGENCY
2810 East Oakland Park Boulevard, Suite 308
Ft Lauderdale, FL 33306 USA
Contact: Robert Stein
FL Lic#: TA 335
T 1 954 561 1226
F 1 954 561 2602
E aveprodrob@aol.com

HART MODELS
915 NE 20th Avenue, 2nd Floor
Ft Lauderdale, FL 33304 USA
Contact: Danielle Hart, President
T 1 954 522 2090
F 1 954 767 8984
E hartmodels@aol.com

Jacques Models
2440 E Commercial Boulevard
Ft Lauderdale, FL 33308 USA
T 1 954 938 7226
F 1 954 938 7228

Models Exchange Talent Agency
2425 E Commercial Boulevard
Ft Lauderdale, FL 33308 USA
T 1 954 491 1014
F 1 954 491 6876

• • • • • • • • • •

S.W. FLORIDA MODELING & TALENT AGENCY
1400 Royal Palm Square Boulevard, Suite 104
Ft Myers, FL 33919 USA
Contact: Stephane Shaffer, Agent
FL Lic#: TA0000535
T 1 941 275 3744
F 1 941 275 9555
W www.swfloridamodeling.com

SUZI'S INTERNATIONAL MODELS
12769 Kedleston Circle
Ft Myers, FL 33912 USA
Contact: Suzi Hosfeld, Director
FL Lic#: TA 0000338
T 1 941 768 8189
T 1 941 377 1537
F 1 877 891 2186

Famous Faces Entertainment & Talent Agency
2013 Harding Street
Hollywood, FL 33020 USA
T 1 954 922 0700
F 1 954 922 0479

MARTIN & DONALDS TALENT AGENCY INC
2131 Hollywood Boulevard, Suite 306
Hollywood, FL 33020 USA
T 1 954 921 2427
F 1 954 921 7635

TOP MODELS INC
1940 Harrison Street, Suite 100A
Hollywood, FL 33020 USA
Contact: Lana Carney
T 1 954 920 0029
F 1 954 920 7929
W www.atopmodel.com
E modlctr@aol.com

Brevard Talent Group Inc
405 Palm Springs Boulevard
Indian Harbor Beach, FL 32937 USA
T 1 321 773 1355
F 1 321 773 1842

MDM Studios
968 Pinetree Drive
Indian Harbor Beach, FL 32937 USA
T 1 321 777 1344

DENISE CAROL MODELS & TALENT
2223 Atlantic Boulevard
Jacksonville, FL 32207 USA
Contact: Suzi Young
FL Lic#: TA000649
T 1 904 399 0824 Studio
T 1 904 398 6306 Clients
W www.denisecarolmodels.com
E denisecarolmodels@ilnk.com

LINBURG MODEL MANAGEMENT
8535 Baymeadows Road, Suite 3-160
Jacksonville, FL 32256-7423 USA
T 1 800 451 5813
F 1 800 236 7071

TAG TALENT
3200 W Oakland Park Boulevard
Lauderdale Lakes, FL 33311 USA
Contact: Tracy Anne George, President
T 1 954 739 6077
T 1 866 824 8748 Toll Free
F 1 954 739 3303
W www.tagtalent.com
E info@tagtalent.com

Longwood

ARIZA TALENT & MODELING AGENCY
1928 Boothe Circle
Longwood, FL 32750 USA
T 1 407 332 0011
F 1 407 332 0206
W www.arizamodelingandtalent.com
E jeffcallender@hotmail.com

Barbizon of Orlando
1917 Boothe Circle, Suite 151
Longwood, FL 32750 USA
T 1 407 331 5558
F 1 407 331 0548

THE DIAMOND AGENCY
204 W Bay Avenue
Longwood, FL 32750 USA
Contact: Marsha McMorrough, Owner
Serving the Orlando-Central Florida Area
T 1 407 830 4040
F 1 407 830 0021
E diamond1000@onebox.com

John Casablancas/MTM
1060 W State Road 434, Suite 136-138
Longwood, FL 32750 USA
T 1 407 265 1500
F 1 407 265 9557

THE REEVE AGENCY
1917 Boothe Circle, Suite 151
Longwood, FL 32750 USA
Contact: Polly Reeve, Vice President
FL Lic#: TA 0000537
T 1 407 331 1784
F 1 407 331 0548

Miami/Miami Beach Area

ANDERSON GREENE ENTERTAINMENT
1210 Washington Avenue, Suite 245
Miami Beach, FL 33139 USA
Contact: Anderson Greene
T 1 305 674 9881
F 1 305 674 9224
E ageof@bellsouth.net

AURA MODEL & TALENT AGENCY
1874 West Avenue, Suite 2A
Miami Beach, FL 33139 USA
T 1 305 673 2400
F 1 305 673 2441

Coconut Grove Model & Talent Agency
3525 Vista Court
Miami, FL 33133 USA
T 1 305 858 3002
F 1 305 285 9377

Elite Miami
1200 Collins Avenue, Suite 207
Miami Beach, FL 33139 USA
T 1 305 674 9500
F 1 305 674 9600

FORD MODELS
311 Lincoln, Suite 205
Miami Beach, FL 33139 USA
T 1 305 534 7200
F 1 305 534 8220

THE GREEN AGENCY INC
1329 Alton Road
Miami Beach, FL 33139 USA
Contact: Tammy Green / Lauren Green
T 1 305 532 9225
F 1 305 532 9334
W www.greenagency.com
E model@greenagency.com

>>

INTERNATIONAL MODELS INC
8415 Coral Way, Suite 205
Miami, FL 33155 USA
Contact: Teresa Portales
FL Lic#: TA 0000347
T 1 305 266 6331
F 1 305 261 7726
E agency@internationalmodelsinc.com

JOHN CASABLANCAS
MTM - MODEL & TALENT MANAGEMENT
10200 NW 25th Street, Suite A-105
Miami, FL 33172 USA
Contact: Angie Lerner, Agency Director
T 1 305 716 0222
F 1 305 716 1165
W www.jcsouthflorida.com
E modelyou@aol.com

IRENE MARIE MANAGEMENT GROUP
728 Ocean Drive
Miami Beach, FL 33139 USA
Contact: Brigitte Heininger, Director/Women's Board
Tino Beretta, Director/Men's Board
T 1 305 672 2929
F 1 305 674 1342
W www.irenemarie.com
E mail@irenemarie.com

KARIN MODELS
846 Lincoln Road, Penthouse
Miami Beach, FL 33139 USA
Contact: Alberto Nota
T 1 305 672 8300 Women
T 1 305 535 8812 Men
F 1 305 531 8330
E alberto@karinmodels.com

MEGA
3618 NE 2nd Avenue (Design District)
Miami, FL 33137 USA
Contact: Marcus Panthera
T 1 305 576 3204
F 1 305 576 9204

M.E.M. MODEL MANAGEMENT
1688 Meridian Avenue, Suite 801
Miami Beach, FL 33139 USA
Contact: Tia Sabourin
T 1 305 534 8866
F 1 305 534 8879
E memmodels@aol.com

MARIANNE MODELS
530 Ocean Drive, Suite 104
Miami Beach, FL 33139 USA
T 1 305 534 2005
F 1 305 534 2048
E marianneagency@worldnet.att.net

MEN'S BOARD MANAGEMENT
WOMEN'S BOARD MANAGEMENT
3618 NE 2nd Avenue (Design District)
Miami, FL 33137 USA
T 1 305 573 1374
F 1 305 438 3715

Models Inc
1000 Lincoln Road, Suite 230
Miami Beach, FL 33139 USA
T 1 305 538 8585
F 1 305 538 3232

NEXT MANAGEMENT • MIAMI
1688 Meridian Avenue, Suite 800
Miami Beach, FL 33139 USA
T 1 305 531 5100
F 1 305 531 7870
W www.nextmodelmanagement.com
***See Ad This Section.**

PAGE PARKES MODELS REP TALENT / PAGE 305
763 Collins Avenue, 4th Floor
Miami Beach, FL 33139 USA
FL Lic#: 278
T 1 305 672 4869
F 1 305 672 1137
W www.page305.com
E women@page305.com
E men@page305.com

PORTFOLIO MODEL MGMT & TALENT GROUP
235 Lincoln Road, Suite 200
Miami Beach, FL 33139 USA
Contact: Philippe L. Medell
T 1 305 534 4210
F 1 305 534 0663
E PTGModels@aol.com

RUNWAYS TALENT GROUP
1688 Meridian Avenue
Miami Beach, FL 33139 USA
T 1 305 673 8245
F 1 305 673 8631

SELECT MODELS • NETWORK MANAGEMENT INC
420 Lincoln Road, Suite 356
Miami Beach, FL 33139 USA
Contact: Cyrus Chamberlain
T 1 305 672 5566
F 1 305 538 7120
W www.selectmdls.com
E selectmdls@aol.com

THE SPORTS BOOK
1688 Meridian Avenue, Suite 500
Miami Beach, FL 33139 USA
T 1 305 531 4005
F 1 305 673 8631

>>

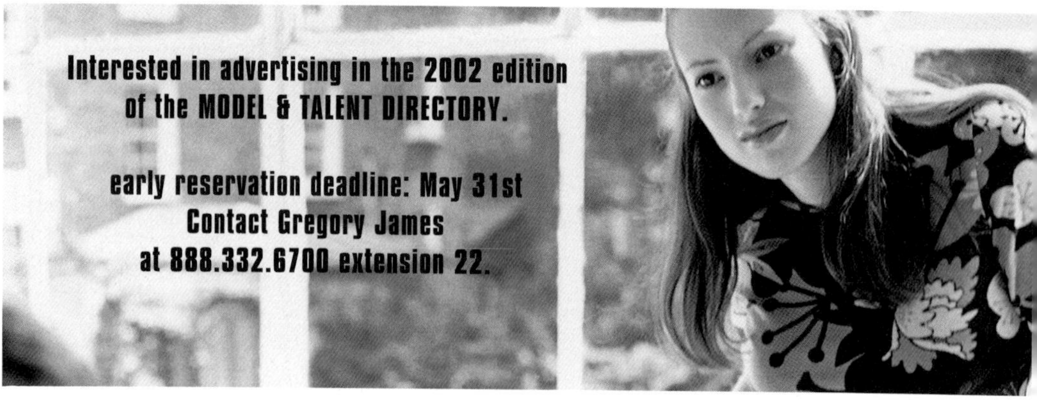
Interested in advertising in the 2002 edition
of the MODEL & TALENT DIRECTORY.
early reservation deadline: May 31st
Contact Gregory James
at 888.332.6700 extension 22.

Star Quality Model & Talent Management
1434 Brickell Avenue
Miami, FL 33131 USA
T 1 305 371 4446
F 1 305 371 4448

Stellar Model & Talent
407 Lincoln Road, Suite 2-K
Miami Beach, FL 33139 USA
T 1 305 672 2217
F 1 305 672 2365

ULTRA MODEL MANAGEMENT
1688 Meridian Avenue, Suite 400
Miami Beach, FL 33139 USA
T 1 305 538 5445
F 1 305 538 7386

UNIQUE CASTING & ASSOCIATES
1613 Alton Road
Miami Beach, FL 33139 USA
T 1 305 532 0226
F 1 305 532 0996
W www.uniquecasting.com
E castmiami@aol.com

WILHELMINA • MIAMI
927 Lincoln Road, Suite 200
Miami Beach, FL 33139 USA
T 1 305 672 9344 Women
T 1 305 674 7203 Men
T 1 305 531 5475 Kids
T 1 305 674 7206 Media
T 1 305 674 7206 Lifestyle
F 1 305 531 8214
***See Ad This Section.**

WORLD OF KIDS
1460 Ocean Drive, Suite 205
Miami Beach, FL 33139 USA
Contact: Debbie Cozzo, Owner
Specializing in Children & Teens; Kid's Stylists
T 1 305 672 5437
F 1 305 672 1989

• • • • • • • • • •

DK Management
3780 Tampa Road, Suite C6
Oldsmar, FL 34677 USA
T 1 813 854 5491
F 1 813 854 4056

John Robert Powers
1170 3rd Street South
Naples, FL 34102 USA
T 1 941 430 0621
F 1 941 430 0618

PROTOCOL MODELS ON THE GULF
5037 Tamiami Trail E
Naples, FL 34113 USA
Contact: Geri Muck, Agent
FL Lic#: TA 0000607
T 1 941 417 1200
F 1 941 417 1207
E protocolmodels@aol.com

Premiere Model Management
502 Canal Street
New Smyrna Beach, FL 32168 USA
T 1 904 427 8829
F 1 904 427 6860

BAILEY'S MODEL MANAGEMENT
1516 E Colonial Drive, Suite 302
Orlando, FL 32803 USA
Contact: Jodi Ledford
T 1 407 894 1910
F 1 407 894 9939
W www.baileysmodel.com
E baileysmodels@aol.com

The Christensen Group
235 Coastline Road
Orlando, FL 32771 USA
T 1 407 302 2272
F 1 407 302 1113

MODELSCOUT INC
651 Rugby Street
Orlando, FL 32804 USA
Contact: Ward Cottrell
Celebrating our 10 Year Anniversary!
T 1 407 420 5888
F 1 407 420 9447
W www.modelscout.com
***See Ad This Section.**

THE MODEL & TALENT GROUP INC
102 Park Street
Safety Harbor, FL 34695 USA
Contact: Pamela Osler-Oleck, Convention Recruiters
T 1 727 669 9119
F 1 727 669 6217
E MODELSGRP@aol.com

STEPHANIE GIBBS MODELS / THE SURF BOARD
1365 South Patrick Drive
Satellite Beach, FL 32937 USA
Contact: Stephanie Gibbs Walker, President
T 1 321 777 9127
F 1 321 777 1512
W www.gibbsmodels.com

Smarter Image Inc
1344 SE McArthur Boulevard
Stuart, FL 34996-4927 USA
T 1 561 225 0898
F 1 561 225 6562

Khara's Set 5 Models & Talent
714 Glenview Road
Tallahassee, FL 32303 USA
T 1 850 224 8500
F 1 850 224 8500

MARSHA DOLL MODELS & PROMOTIONS INC
2131 Orleans Drive
Tallahassee, FL 32308 USA
Contact: Marsha Doll-Faulkenberry, President
T 1 850 656 2600
F 1 850 656 2600
E marshadoll@aol.com

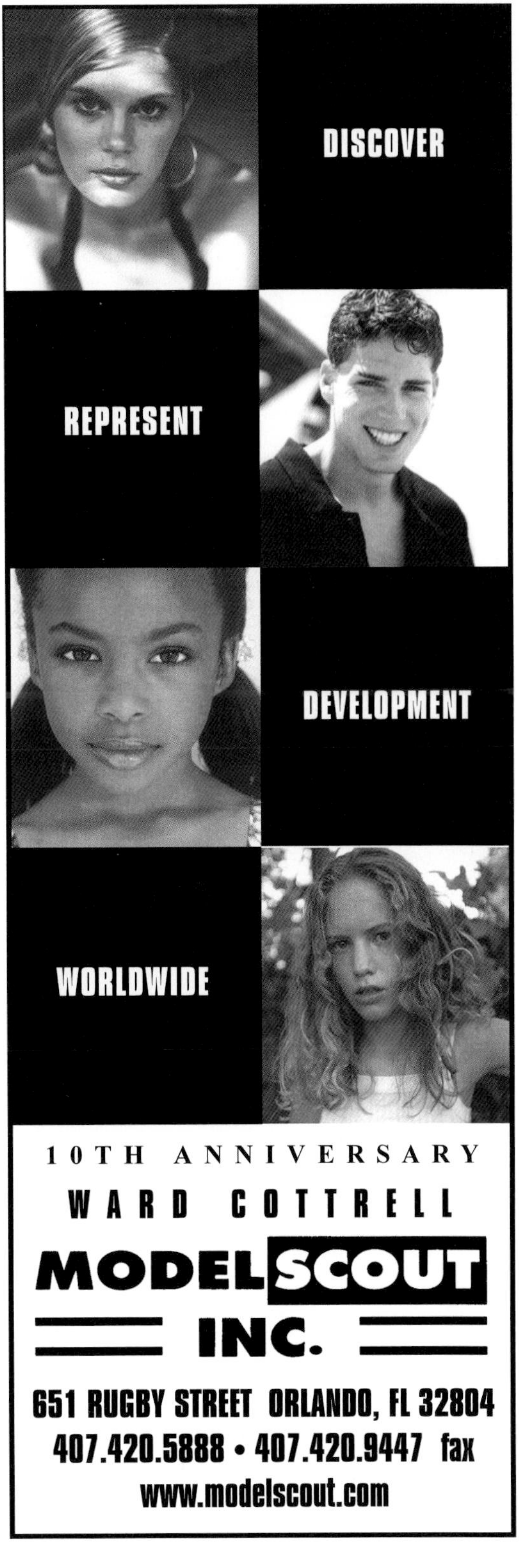

FLORIDA

Tampa

ALEXA MODEL & TALENT MANAGEMENT INC
4100 West Kennedy, Suite 228
Tampa, FL 33609 USA
Contact: Susan Schwabinger
T 1 813 289 8020
F 1 813 286 8281
W www.alexamodels.com
E alexa@dreamport.com

BOOM MODEL & TALENT AGENCY
13012 North Dale Mabry, Suite B
Tampa, FL 33618 USA
Contact: Di Paulson
FL Lic#: TA0000475
T 1 813 264 1373
F 1 813 264 7213
W www.boommodel.com
E boommodel@aol.com
***See Ad This Section.**

FIRST IMPRESSIONS INC
41 Davis Boulevard
Tampa, FL 33606 USA
Contact: Joann Torretta, Owner/Director
Members of Assn. of Image Consultant Int'l
& The Fashion Group
T 1 813 251 1008
F 1 813 251 3384
E TorrettaFl@aol.com

Independent Castings Inc
8313 W Hillsborough Avenue
Tampa, FL 33615 USA
T 1 813 884 8335
F 1 813 884 9422

John Casablancas/MTM
5215 W Laurel Street, Suite 110
Tampa, FL 33607 USA
T 1 813 289 8564
F 1 813 289 2746

look
MODEL · TALENT
AGENCY
TA# 0000567

LOOK MODEL & TALENT AGENCY
1320 E 6th Avenue, Ybor City
Tampa, FL 33605 USA
Contact: Steve Benz
T 1 813 242 4400
F 1 813 241 4500
W www.lookagency.com
E lookmodl@gte.net

SHOWBIZ KIDZ! DEVELOPMENT CENTER
4237 Henderson Blvd
Tampa, FL 33629 USA
Contact: M. Susan Walls
Consultation/Workshops for ages 4-17 Actors • Dancers • Singers • Print Models • Vocal Coaching • Pageant Preparation • Pilot Season-LA
T 1 813 639 0922
F 1 813 639 1164
W www.showbizkidz.org
E prinkey@mindspring.com

• • • • • • • • • •

CHRISTI KNIGHT FASHION PRODUCTIONS & TALENT AGENCY
80 Royal Palm Boulevard, Suite 402
Vero Beach, FL 32963 USA
Contact: Christi Knight
FL Lic.# TA0000595
T 1 561 978 7997
F 1 561 569 1455
E ckfp@usa.com

Nouveau Models Intl
2600 Broadway, Suite A
W Palm Beach, FL 33407 USA
T 1 561 659 3656
F 1 561 832 9024

Sarah Parker Model & Talent
410 Datura Street
W Palm Beach, FL 33401 USA
T 1 561 655 4400
F 1 561 655 1222

Azuree Talent Agency Inc
140 N Orlando Avenue, Suite 120
Winter Park, FL 32789 USA
T 1 407 629 5025
F 1 407 629 0122

The Hurt Agency
400 N New York Avenue
Winter Park, FL 32789 USA
T 1 407 740 5700
F 1 407 740 0929

MODEL & TALENT AGENCIES

GEORGIA

The Voice Casting Network
8950 Laurel Way
Alpharetta, GA 30202 USA
T 1 770 518 9855
F 1 770 518 9853

Atlanta

ABOUT FACES MODELS AND TALENT
3391 Peachtree Road, Suite 410
Atlanta, GA 30326 USA
Contact: Lesa Rummell La Force
T 1 404 233 2006
F 1 404 237 2578
W www.aboutfacesmt.com

A-LINE MODEL & TALENT MARKETING
120 W Wieuca Road, Suite 103
Atlanta, GA 30342 USA
Contact: Karen Troncalli, Director
T 1 404 459 8933
F 1 404 459 8936
W www.a-linemodels.com

AMC Inc
250 Spring Street NW
Atlanta, GA 30303 USA
T 1 404 220 2833
F 1 404 220 2813

Arlene Wilson Model Management
887 W Marietta Street NW
Atlanta, GA 30318 USA
T 1 404 876 8555
F 1 404 876 9043

Atlanta's Young Faces / Look Model Mgmt
6075 Roswell Road NE, Suite 118
Atlanta, GA 30328 USA
T 1 404 255 3080
F 1 404 255 3173

AXIS MODEL MANAGEMENT INC
120 W Wieuca Road, Suite 107
Atlanta, GA 30342 USA
Contact: Douglas Hill, President
T 1 404 459 0881
F 1 404 459 0884
W www.axismodels.com
E axismodels@mindspring.com

BABES 'N BEAUS
4757 Canton Road, Suite 107
Atlanta, GA 30066 USA
Contact: Linda D. Rutledge, Director
T 1 770 928 5832
F 1 770 928 3701

BARBIZON OF ATLANTA
3340 Peachtree Road, Tower Walk
Atlanta, GA 30326 USA
Contact: Michael Bartolacci
T 1 404 261 7332
F 1 404 261 7362
W www.modelingschools.com
E mrbarto@aol.com

Click Models
79 Poplar Street, Suite B
Atlanta, GA 30303 USA
T 1 404 261 7332
F 1 404 261 7362

ELITE MODEL MANAGEMENT
1708 Peachtree Street NW, Suite 210
Atlanta, GA 30309 USA
T 1 404 872 7444
F 1 404 874 1526
W www.eliteatlanta.com
E elitemodels@eliteatlanta.com

GALAXY MODEL & TALENT AGENCY
3340 Peachtree Road, Tower Walk
Atlanta, GA 30326 USA
Contact: Michael Bartolacci
T 1 404 261 7332
F 1 404 261 7362
E mrbarto@aol.com

John Robert Powers
1197 Peechtree Street, Suite 555
Atlanta, GA 30361 USA
T 1 404 877 1155

>>

KIDDIN' AROUND / REAL PEOPLE MODELS & TALENT
1479 Spring Street
Atlanta, GA 30309 USA
Contact: Eva Stancil, President
T 1 404 872 8582
F 1 404 872 8590
E kiddin@mindspring.com

L'AGENCE
5901C Peachtree Dunwoody Road, Suite 60
Atlanta, GA 30328 USA
Contact: Gretta Cook • Mark Cook • Senia Cook
T 1 770 396 9015
T 1 770 396 7657 TV
F 1 770 391 0927
W www.lagencemodels.com

MADISON AGENCY
426 Marietta Street NW, Suite 410
Atlanta, GA 30313 USA
Contact: Teresa Kellar
T 1 678 302 8650
F 1 678 302 8654
E MadisonAtl@aol.com

SLAMM MODEL MANAGEMENT
233 Mitchell Street, Suite 300
Atlanta, GA 30303 USA
Contact: Rodney Harris
T 1 404 302 9344
F 1 404 302 9354

• • • • • • • • • •

MICHELLE JAMES
MODELING PRODUCTIONS
467 Highland Avenue
Augusta, GA 30909 USA
Contact: Sharon Speights
T 1 706 738 7707
W www.michellejames.com
E sspeight@michellejames.com

MODEL PRODUCTIONS MODEL & TALENT AGENCY
3604 Verandah Drive
Augusta, GA 30909 USA
Contact: Bill & Carolyn Waldbueser
T 1 706 731 9889
F 1 706 731 9890

Burns Agency
3800 Brettonwood Road
Decatur, GA 30032 USA
T 1 336 744 5037
F 1 336 744 5039

MADEMOISELLE MODELS
2901 University Avenue, Suite 16
Columbus, GA 31907 USA
Contact: Deborah L. Hatcher, Owner
Host of the Worldwide Modeling Convention
T 1 706 561 9449
F 1 706 561 9741
W www.mademoisellemodels.com
E beamodel@aol.com

DYSART MODELING/TALENT/CASTING
4566 Oxford Drive
Evans, GA 30809 USA
Contact: Evelyn Dysart
T 1 706 868 7221
T 1 706 650 1080
C 1 706 564 7171
F 1 706 868 8232
W www.dysartagency.com
E evelyn@dysartagency.com

Modeling Images
2106 Chatou Place
Kennesaw, GA 30152 USA
T 1 770 919 8285

ATLANTA'S EDGE MODEL MANAGEMENT
360 Killian Hill Road, Suite F-2
Lilburn, GA 30047 USA
Contact: Bobby Duerr / Angela Braden
T 1 770 806 1223
F 1 770 806 1932
E edgemodelmngt@mindspring.com

LORREN & MACY'S MODELING SCHOOL
& TALENT AGENCY
235 Riverbend Mall SW, Suite 235
Rome, GA 30161 USA
Contact: Judy Lorren-Fincher
T 1 706 235 1175
F 1 706 291 3740
F 1 706 235 1175

Glyn Kennedy Agency
975 Hunterhill Drive
Roswell, GA 30075 USA
T 1 678 461 4444
F 1 678 461 4422

Millie Lewis Modeling & Finishing School
7011 Hodgson Memorial Drive
Savannah, GA 31406 USA
T 1 912 354 9525
F 1 912 353 9146

Talent Source
107 East Hall Street
Savannah, GA 31401 USA
T 1 912 232 9390
F 1 912 232 8213

Eileen's Models
917 Williamsburg Drive
Valdosta, GA 31602 USA
T 1 912 244 2755

MODEL & TALENT AGENCIES

HAWAII

JJ Modeling Agency & Productions
98-021 JJP Lane/OFF Highway, 2nd Floor
Aiea, Oahu, HI 96701 USA
T 1 808 486 1656
F 1 808 486 1657

ADR MODEL & TALENT AGENCY
419 Waiakamilo Road, Suite 204
Honolulu, HI 96817 USA
Contact: Ryan K. Brown, President
T 1 808 842 1313
F 1 808 842 1186
W www.adragency.com
E info@adragency.com

E.L. MODELS INTERNATIONAL
60 N Beretania Street, Suite 2802
Honolulu, HI 96817-4761 USA
Contact: Emily Lopez
T 1 808 550 2656
F 1 808 550 2803
W www.elmodels.com
E elmodels@elmodels.com

KATHY MULLER TALENT & MODELING AGENCY
619 Kapahulu Avenue, PH
Honolulu, HI 96815 USA
Contact: Ann Mata, Agency Director
Great Talent, Print, Commercials, Film.
Private locations available for all types of shoots, weddings & functions.
T 1 808 737 7917
F 1 808 734 3026
E kma@panworld.net

MORE MODELS & TALENT
1311 Kapiolani Blvd, Suite 605
Honolulu, HI 96814 USA
Contact: Sri or Ruz
T 1 808 596 7717
F 1 808 596 7718
E moremodl@lava.net
***See Ad This Section.**

≫

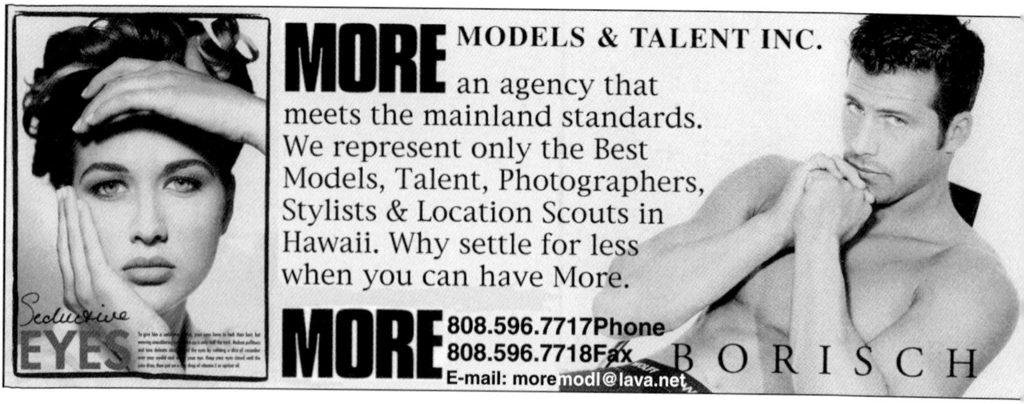

Premiere Models & Talent
1441 Kapiolani Boulevard, Suite 1206
Honolulu, HI 96814 USA
T 1 808 955 6511
F 1 808 955 9385

Ruth Woodhall Talent Agency
411 Hoberon Lane, Suite 3306
Honolulu, HI 96815 USA
T 1 808 947 3307
F 1 808 947 3307

Susan Page's Modeling & Talent
1441 Kapiolani Boulevard, Suite 1206
Honolulu, HI 96814 USA
T 1 808 955 2271
F 1 808 955 9385

V TALENT & MODEL MANAGEMENT
2153 N King Street, Suite 323-A
Honolulu, HI 96819 USA
Contact: Vilma Cafirma Tucay, President/Owner
A Screen Actors Guild Franchise Agency
T 1 808 842 0881
T 1 888 55V 6483
F 1 808 848 0991
W www.vtalentmgmt.com
E vtalent@hawaii.rr.com

Focus International Model & Talent Agency
74-5615 Luhia Street, Suite A2
Kailua Kona, HI 96740 USA
T 1 808 323 3333
F 1 808 882 7511

CHAMELEON TALENT AGENCY
P.O. Box 959
Kihei, HI 96753 USA
Contact: Cynthia Clark, President
T 1 808 879 7817
F 1 808 875 9197
W www.chameleontalent.com
E talent@aloha.net

CIA MODELS MANAGEMENT & PRODUCTIONS
41-846 Laumilo Street
Waimanalo, HI 96795 USA
Contact: Kim Medeiros, President
T 1 808 259 7914
F 1 808 259 8913
E cia808@earthlink.net

MODEL & TALENT AGENCIES

IDAHO

BLANCHE B. EVANS SCHOOL/AGENCY INTERNATIONAL
4311 Audubon Place
Boise, ID 83705 USA
Contact: Blanche B. Evans
T 1 208 344 5380
F 1 208 344 5380

METCALF MODELING & TALENT AGENCY
1851 S Century Way, Suite 3
Boise, ID 83709 USA
Contact: Bonnie Metcalf, Owner
Brian Bair, Agency Director
Shaun Ferguson, Asst. Agency Director
T 1 208 378 8777
T 1 208 378 8838
F 1 208 327 0653
E metcalfagt@aol.com

MODEL & TALENT AGENCIES

ILLINOIS

Ambassador Talent Agents, Inc
333 North Michigan Avenue, Suite 910
Chicago, IL 60601 USA
T 1 312 641 3491
F 1 312 641 3773

ARIA MODEL & TALENT MANAGEMENT
1017 West Washington, Suite 2C
Chicago, IL 60607 USA
T 1 312 243 9400
F 1 312 243 9020
W www.ariamodel.com

Arlene Wilson Model Management
430 W Erie Street
Chicago, IL 60610 USA
T 1 312 573 0200
F 1 312 573 0046

ASAP MODELS/TALENT PROMOTION LTD
P.O. Box 408080
Chicago, IL 60640 USA
Contact: Barre Lerner
Promotions, Trade Shows, Runway, Film, Print, Conventions
T 1 773 755 0000
F 1 773 348 2923
E ASAPMODPR@aol.com

Bea Corey Management
1030 N State Street, Suite 36C
Chicago, IL 60610 USA
T 1 312 604 4602
F 1 702 228 5079

BEST FACES OF CHICAGO
1152 North La Salle, Suite F
Chicago, IL 60610 USA
Contact: Judy Mudd, Owner
T 1 312 944 3009
F 1 312 944 7006
W www.bestfacesofchicago.com
E bestfaceschicago@aol.com

BMG WORLDWIDE MODEL MANAGEMENT
314 W Institute Place, Loft 2W
Chicago, IL 60610 USA
Contact: Gregory Brown, President
T 1 312 664 1516
F 1 312 664 1558
E Eyescout@aol.com

CLASSIC MODEL AND TALENT MANAGEMENT
225 W Washington, Suite 2200
Chicago, IL 60606 USA
Contact: Kathy Nedved
T 1 312 419 7192
F 1 312 419 7151
W www.rivint.com/classic
E classic@rivint.com
***See Ad This Section.**

ELITE MODEL MANAGEMENT
58 West Huron
Chicago, IL 60610 USA
TV/Film Affiliate: Stewart Talent
T 1 312 943 3226
F 1 312 943 2590
W www.elitechicago.com
E elitemodels@elitechicago.com

Emila Lorence, Ltd
325 W Huron Street
Chicago, IL 60610 USA
T 1 312 787 2033
F 1 312 787 5239

FORD CHICAGO
641 W Lake Street, Suite 402
Chicago, IL 60661 USA
T 1 312 707 9000
F 1 312 707 8515

Geddes Agency
1633 N Halsted Street
Chicago, IL 60614 USA
T 1 312 787 8333
F 1 312 787 6677

Harrise Davidson Talent Agency
1532 N Milwaukee Avenue
Chicago, IL 60622 USA
T 1 773 384 7300
F 1 773 384 7900

>>

HYPE MODEL MANAGEMENT
954 W Washington
Chicago, IL 60607 USA
Contact: Bruno Abate
T 1 312 243 8547
F 1 312 243 8571
W www.hypemodel.com
E hypemodels@aol.com

JOHN ROBERT POWERS
27 E Monroe Street
Chicago, IL 60603 USA
Contact: Joseph Durkin
T 1 312 726 1404
F 1 312 726 8019
E jrp@interaccess.com

Models Unlimited
415 N LaSalle, Suite 202
Chicago, IL 60610 USA
T 1 312 329 1001
F 1 312 329 2003

Nouvelle Talent Management
P.O. Box 578100
Chicago, IL 60657 USA
T 1 312 944 1133
F 1 312 944 2298

PLATINUM MODEL MANAGEMENT
633 S Plymouth Court, Suite 204
Chicago, IL 60605 USA
T 1 312 588 1840
F 1 312 588 0054
W www.platinummodelmgmt.com
E platinummodel2@aol.com

Salazar & Navas, Inc
760 N Ogden Avenue, Suite 2200
Chicago, IL 60622 USA
T 1 312 666 1677
F 1 312 666 1681

SCOUT OFFICE • WORLDWIDE AGENCY REPRESENTATION
314 W Institute Place, Loft 2W
Chicago, IL 60610 USA
Contact: Gregory Brown, President
T 1 312 664 1609
F 1 312 664 1558
E Eyescout@aol.com

Shirley Hamilton, Inc
333 E Ontairo, Suite 302B
Chicago, IL 60611 USA
T 1 312 787 4700
F 1 312 787 8456

STEWART TALENT
58 W Huron Street
Chicago, IL 60610 USA
T 1 312 943 3131
F 1 312 943 5107
W www.stewarttalent.com

Talent Group Inc
1228 W Wilson Avenue
Chicago, IL 60640 USA
T 1 773 561 8814
F 1 773 728 5896

WY INTERNATIONAL MODELS INC
162 N Franklin Street, Suite 401A
Chicago, IL 60606 USA
Contact: Yi Wang
T 1 312 849 9190
F 1 312 849 9508
W www.wymodels.com
E WYIModels@aol.com

• • • • • • • • • •

Joy Dickens Productions
9236 N Springfield
Evanston, IL 60203 USA
T 1 847 677 2643
F 1 847 677 2654

Norman Schucart Enterprises
1417 Green Bay Road
Highland Pk, IL 60035 USA
T 1 847 433 1113
F 1 847 433 1113

North Shore Talent Inc
454 Peterson Road
Libertyville, IL 60048 USA
T 1 847 816 1811
F 1 847 816 1717

SHAWNEE STUDIOS INC
MODEL & TALENT MANAGEMENT
102 W Main Street
Mt Olive, IL 62069 USA
Contact: Shawnee
T 1 217 999 2522
T 1 877 675 9755 Out of State 800#
F 1 217 999 2214
W www.shawneestudios.com
E shawnee@mt-olive.com

McBlaine & Associates
805 W Touhy Avenue
Park Ridge, IL 60068 USA
T 1 847 823 9763
F 1 847 823 1253

Barbizon
1051 Perimeter Drive, Suite 950
Schaumburg, IL 60173 USA
T 1 847 240 4200
F 1 847 240 4212

ROYAL MODEL MANAGEMENT
1051 Perimeter Drive
Schaumburg, IL 60173 USA
Contact: Anne Emmrich, Director
T 1 847 240 4215
F 1 847 240 4212
***See Ad This Section.**

CLAIRE MODEL & TALENT
P.O. Box 1028
Wheeling, IL 60090 USA
Contact: Clarice Rosenstock
Serving Chicagoland Area for
Promotions & Trade Shows
T 1 847 459 4242
F 1 847 459 0001
E clarmdl@aol.com

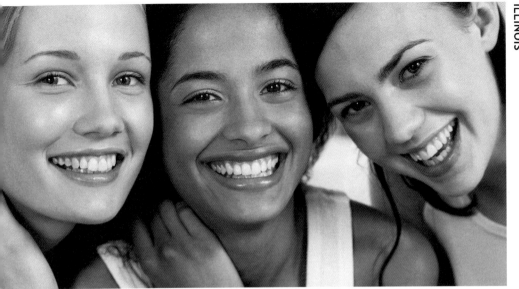

MODEL & TALENT AGENCIES

INDIANA

SUPER! MODELS INTERNATIONAL
14420 Cherry Tree Road
Carmel, IN 46033 USA
Contact: Jessy Henderson / Ro Pettiner
T 1 317 846 4321

Charmaine School & Model Agency
3538 Stellhorn Road
Ft Wayne, IN 46815 USA
T 1 219 485 8421
F 1 219 485 1873

AAA Modeling Agency
11777 Park Lane North
Granger, IN 46530 USA
T 1 219 247 9052
F 1 219 247 9067

EVELYN LAHAIE MODELING
P.O. Box 614
Hobart, IN 46342-0614 USA
Contact: Evelyn Lahaie
T 1 219 942 4670
F 1 219 733 2318

Helen Wells Agency
401 Pennsylvania Parkway, Suite 101
Indianapolis, IN 46280 USA
T 1 317 843 5363
F 1 317 843 5364

ON TRACK MODELING INC
77 South Girlschool Road, Suite 105
Indianapolis, IN 46231 USA
T 1 317 381 9384
F 1 317 381 9386
***See Ad This Section.**

MODEL & TALENT AGENCIES

IOWA

Model Consultants
2625 SE 18th Street
Des Moines, IA 50320 USA
T 1 515 244 5500

UNIVERSAL MODEL & TALENT MANAGEMENT
10095 Hickman Court, Suite 3
Des Moines, IA 50325 USA
Contact: Sean Kisner
T 1 515 278 5432
F 1 515 278 6622
E universalmtm@aol.com

Genesis
1180 1/2 7th Avenue
Marion, IA 52302 USA
T 1 319 373 3515
F 1 319 373 3522

Corrine Shover Model School Agency & Marketing
326 North Walnut
Monticello, IA 52310 USA
T 1 319 465 5507
F 1 319 465 5507

AVANT MODELING & TALENT
10546 Justin Drive
Urbandale, IA 50322 USA
Contact: Tina DePhillips, Owner
Bonnie Metcalf, General Manager/International Agent
T 1 515 255 0297
F 1 515 255 1179

MODEL & TALENT AGENCIES

KANSAS

The Agency, Models & Talent
12115 W 82nd Terrace
Lenexa, KS 66215 USA
T 1 913 342 8382
F 1 913 894 0238

CAREER IMAGES MODEL & TALENT AGENCY
8519 Lathrop Avenue
Kansas City, KS 66109 USA
Contact: Raymond La Pietra, Owner
T 1 913 334 2200
F 1 913 334 1990
W www.careerimages.com
E modelman@careerimages.com

HOFFMAN INTERNATIONAL
6705 W 91st Street
Overland Park, KS 66212 USA
Contact: Kim Hoffman, AFTRA
T 1 913 642 9212
F 1 913 642 9229
W www.hoffmanmodels.com
E info@hoffmanmodels.com

IMAGE DEVELOPMENT GROUP
10967 Gillette Street
Overland Park, KS 66210 USA
Contact: Debra Fox
T 1 913 317 8141
TF 1 888 262 6368
F 1 913 317 8149
W www.imagedevelopmentgroup.com
E dfox@imagedevelopmentgroup.com

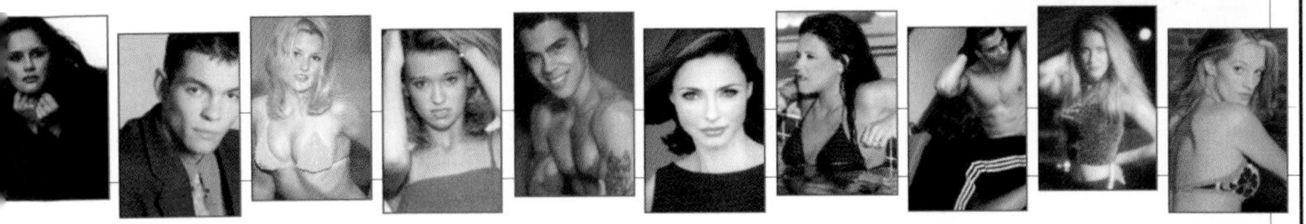

FOCUS MODEL TALENT MANAGEMENT
155 N Market, Suite 140
Wichita, KS 67202 USA
Contact: Maxine Gray, Owner
T 1 316 264 3100
F 1 316 264 3100
W www.focusmtm.com
E focusmtm@hotmail.com

Models & Images
1619 North Rock Road
Wichita, KS 67206 USA
T 1 316 634 2777
F 1 316 634 0121

MODEL & TALENT AGENCIES

KENTUCKY

Alix Adams Agency
9813 Merioneth Drive
Jeffersontown, KY 40299 USA
T 1 502 266 6990
F 1 502 266 7228

IMAGES MODEL AGENCY
163 E Reynolds Road
Lexington, KY 40517 USA
Contact: Janie Olmstead Head, Owner/Director
T 1 606 273 2301
F 1 606 271 3293
W www.imagesmodelagency.com

VOGUE OF LEXINGTON MODEL & TALENT AGENCY INC
1300 New Circle Road, Suite 112
Lexington, KY 40555-5346 USA
Contact: Sarah Bennett Khan
T 1 859 254 4582
F 1 859 254 1137
E voguelex@gateway.com

COSMO MODEL & TALENT
7410 Lagrange Road, Suite 204
Louisville, KY 40222 USA
Contact: Dona Downing, Owner
T 1 502 425 8000
F 1 502 426 2142
W www.cosmomodelsandtalent.com

>>

KENTUCKY

MJK STUDIO • MODEL & TALENT AGENCY
414 Baxter Avenue
Louisville, KY 40204 USA
Contact: Chris Kaufman, Owner/Director
T 1 502 585 4152
F 1 502 589 5502
E mjkmodels@mindspring.com

DIAMOND MODEL & TALENT AGENCY
1195A South Main Street
Madisonville, KY 42431 USA
Contact: Penny Giardinella, Director
T 1 270 821 0600
F 1 270 821 0660
W www.diamondmodels.com
E diamond@diamondmodels.com

AMERICA'S TOP MODELS
58 Public Square
Somerset, KY 42501 USA
T 1 606 451 1778
F 1 606 451 8299

MODEL & TALENT AGENCIES

LOUISIANA

OPEN RANGE MANAGEMENT INC
9185 Wynnewood
Baton Rouge, LA 70815 USA
Contact: Brenda Netzberger
T 1 225 216 2424
F 1 225 926 9515
W www.openrangemgmt.com
E openrange@bellsouth.net

STAGE 2000 MODEL & TALENT CENTER
8133 Royalwood Drive
Baton Rouge, LA 70806 USA
Contact: Ron Randell, Director
T 1 225 216 9195
F 1 225 927 1644
W www.stage2000.net
E randell@premier.net

John Casablancas Model & Career Center
880 West Commerce Road, Suite 103
Harahan, LA 70123 USA
T 1 504 818 1000
F 1 504 734 8723

MTP/Model & Talent Plus
880 West Commerce Road, Suite 103
Harahan, LA 70123 USA
T 1 504 818 1800
F 1 504 734 8723

Aboutfaces Model & Talent Management
423 Jefferson Street, P.O. Box 92243
Lafayette, LA 70501 USA
T 1 337 235 3223
F 1 337 235 3111

IMAGES MODEL & TALENT AGENCY
200 Polk Street, Suite 101
Lafayette, LA 70501 USA
Contact: Simone Steen, President
T 1 337 291 2913
F 1 337 291 2973
E 511images@bellsouth.net

Glamour Modeling & Talent
P.O. Box 1526
Meraux, LA 70075-1526 USA
T 1 504 279 7313
F 1 504 279 7313

New Orleans

ABA Convention Models
4518 Magazine Street
New Orleans, LA 70115 USA
T 1 504 895 2000
F 1 504 891 7177

ABOUTFACES MODEL & TALENT MANAGEMENT
929 Julia Street, 2nd Floor
New Orleans, LA 70113 USA
Contact: Tracey Dundas
T 1 504 522 3030
T 1 800 504 7080 Voice Mail
T 1 318 235 3223 Lafayette Office
F 1 504 522 0850
E aboutfacesmtm@aol.com

DEL CORRAL MODEL & TALENT AGENCY INC
The Talent Centre, 130 S Telemachus
New Orleans, LA 70119 USA
Contact: Kenneth del Corral, President
T 1 504 486 6335
F 1 504 486 3020
W www.angelfire.com/la/delcorral/index.html
E Agencyl@aol.com

AMEAGENCY.COM INC
4004 Magazine Street
New Orleans, LA 70115 USA
Contact: Lee MacKenzie
FULL SERVICE MODEL & TALENT AGENCY
T 1 800 458 9112
T 1 504 891 2001
F 1 504 891 7177
W www.fameagency.com
E info@fameagency.com

METRO MODEL & TALENT MANAGEMENT
201 St. Charles Avenue, Suite 2587
New Orleans, LA 70170 USA
Contact: Andrew Castro / Bryan Metoyer
T 1 504 897 6686
F 1 504 891 0826
E Metromtm@aol.com

Model Masters Inc
P.O. Box 820134
New Orleans, LA 70182-0134 USA
T 1 504 288 3315
F 1 504 283 6190

New Orleans Model/Talent Agency
1347 Magazine Street
New Orleans, LA 70130 USA
T 1 504 525 0100
F 1 504 525 6621

VICTOR'S INTERNATIONAL MODEL & TALENT MANAGEMENT
618 North Carrollton Avenue
New Orleans, LA 70119 USA
Contact: Victor Schmitt, President
T 1 504 484 7255
F 1 504 484 7293
E vicintl@bellsouth.net

FRANCE INTERNATIONAL
1510 Fairfield Avenue
Shreveport, LA 71104 USA
Contact: Cynthia Jones-France
Also represent photographers & make-up artists.
T 1 318 219 3600
F 1 318 219 3700

THE MICHAEL TURNEY AGENCY
1805 Line Avenue
Shreveport, LA 71101 USA
Contact: Michael Turney / Julianna Woodruff
T 1 318 221 2628
F 1 318 226 0971
W www.MichaelTurneyAgency.com

MODEL & TALENT AGENCIES

MAINE

Maine Talent Source
Point Road, Box 814A
Belgrade, ME 04917 USA
T 1 207 495 2143
F 1 207 495 2446

MODEL & TALENT AGENCIES

MARYLAND

NOVA MODELS INC
2120 N Charles Street
Baltimore, MD 21218 USA
Contact: Christian David / Michael Evans
T 1 410 752 6682
F 1 410 752 5053
***See Ad This Section.**

Savvy Model Management
4315 Belair Road, Suite D
Baltimore, MD 21206 USA
T 1 410 488 5133
F 1 410 488 4808

>>

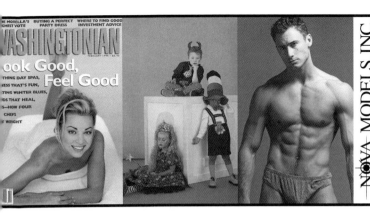

MARYLAND

Scappatori Model Management
6600 York Street, Suite 105
Baltimore, MD 21212 USA
T 1 800 451 5813
F 1 800 236 7071

I'M OUTTA HERE ENTERTAINMENT
1300 Mercantile Lane, Suite 100-D
Largo, MD 20774 USA
Contact: Jeannie Jones
T 1 301 386 7886
F 1 301 386 7885
E ImOuttaHereEnt@aol.com

ANNAPOLIS AGENCY / KIDZ IN THE BIZ INC
P.O. Box 1753
Pasadena, MD 21123 USA
Contact: Cory Cortina, Booker
T 1 410 647 4600
F 1 410 647 5313
W www.kidzinthebiz.com

MODEL & TALENT AGENCIES

MASSACHUSETTS

Boston

BARBIZON MODEL & TALENT AGENCY
607 Boylston Street
Boston, MA 02116 USA
Contact: Claire Williams
T 1 617 266 6980
F 1 617 266 6092

Boston Casting
JFK, P.O. Box 9067
Boston, MA 02114 USA
T 1 617 437 6600
F 1 617 437 6677

Click
125 Newbury Street, Suite 5A
Boston, MA 02116 USA
T 1 617 266 1100
F 1 617 437 6214

COPLEY SEVEN / JO MODEL MANAGEMENT
P.O. Box 535
Boston, MA 02117 USA
Contact: Jo Somers
T 1 617 267 4444
F 1 617 423 3036
W www.copleyseven.com
E info@copleyseven.com

DYNASTY INTERNATIONAL MODEL & TALENT AGENCY INC
207 Newbury Street
Boston MA 02116 USA
Contact: Ginger & Joe Freeman, Directors
T 1 617 536 7900
F 1 617 536 7728
W www.dynastymodels.com
E dyn@dynastymodels.com

FORD MODEL MANAGEMENT INC
297 Newbury Street
Boston, MA 02115 USA
Contact: Candy Ford
Men, Women, Kids • Print, Runway, Promo
T 1 617 266 6939
F 1 617 266 4330
W www.candyford.com
E Ford@gis.net

IMAGE MAKERS
77 Franklin Street, 3rd Floor
Boston, MA 02110 USA
T 1 617 482 3622
F 1 617 482 3624

JOHN ROBERT POWERS
125 Broad Street
Boston, MA 02110 USA
Contact: Arlene Pedjoe, Owner
T 1 617 946 0508
F 1 617 946 2903
W www.johnrobertpowers.com

MAGGIE INC
35 Newbury Street
Boston, MA 02116 USA
Contact: Maggie
T 1 617 536 2639
F 1 617 536 0651
E maggiecorp@aol.com

MODEL CLUB INC CHILDREN
115 Newbury Street, 2nd Floor
Boston, MA 02116 USA
Contact: Ed Sliney
Call for Agency Book...
Will Overnight Express Immediately.
T 1 617 247 9020
F 1 617 247 9262
W www.modelclubinc.com
E modelclubinc@cybercom.net

THE MODELS GROUP
374 Congress Street, Suite 305
Boston, MA 02210 USA
Contact: Kathy Baxter
T 1 617 426 4711
F 1 617 426 6096
E themodelsgroup@juno.com

eautiful Kids Inc
29 Shattuck Road
Hadley, MA 01035 USA
T 1 413 549 2006
F 1 413 549 1974

GENCY ROYALE MODELING
65 Clinton Street, 3rd Floor
Malden, MA 02148 USA
Contact: Sandra Cottreau
T 1 781 397 0993
F 1 781 324 4875
W www.agencyroyale.com
E agencyroyale@agencyroyale.com

ITM • MODEL & TALENT MANAGEMENT
P.O. Box 600646
Newtonville, MA 02460-0646 USA
Contact: Amy Lampinen
T 1 617 969 3555
F 1 617 969 4582

Boston Agency for Children
380 Broadway
Somerville, MA 02145 USA
T 1 617 666 0900
F 1 617 623 2581

The Cameo Agency/Cameo Kids
49 River Street, Suite 1
Waltham, MA 02453-8345 USA
T 1 781 647 8300
F 1 781 647 8303

ANN MILLER MANAGEMENT
P.O. Box 2058
Westfield, MA 01085 USA
Contact: Tim Harrington
Covering MA, CT & Cape Cod for Promotions, Print, Casting & Field Managers.
T 1 413 221 4150
T 1 888 712 0248 Pager
E AMillerM@aol.com

JOHN ROBERT POWERS
390 Main Street
Worcester, MA 01608 USA
Contact: Arlene Pedjoe
T 1 508 753 6343
F 1 508 791 0331
W www.johnrobertpowers.com
E jrp84worc@email.msn.com

MODEL & TALENT AGENCIES

MICHIGAN

Ta-Dah Productions
2737 W 12 Mile Road
Berkley, MI 48072 USA
T 1 248 548 2324
F 1 248 548 6380

THE TALENT SHOP
30100 Telegraph Road, Suite 116
Bingham Farms, MI 48025 USA
Contact: Jackie Kagan, President/CEO
T 1 248 644 4877
F 1 248 644 0331
W www.thetalentshopgroup.com
E info@thetalentshopgroup.com

PRODUCTIONS PLUS / NATIONWIDE TALENT & CASTING AGENCY
30600 Telegraph Road, Suite 2156
Birmingham, MI 48025 USA
Contact: Margery Krevsky, President or DJ Wallace, Director of Special Events
T 1 248 644 5566
F 1 248 644 6072
W www.productions-plus.com
E m_krevsky@productions-plus.com
E dj@productions-plus.com

SUCCESS MODEL & TALENT AGENCY
101 Brookside Lane, Suite N
Brighton, MI 48116 USA
Contact: Dennis Wm. McVittie Sr
T 1 810 220 5902
F 1 810 220 5907

JOHN CASABLANCAS / MTM MODEL & TALENT MANAGEMENT
45185 Joy Road, Suite 101
Canton, MI 48187 USA
Contact: Keith Strickland
T 1 734 455 0700
F 1 734 455 2156
E mtmdetroit@yahoo.com

SHORTDWARF.COM
1295 Stoll Road
Dewitt, MI 48820-8646 USA
Contact: Chuck Hart, Agent
T 1 517 371 2225
F 1 517 371 2725
W www.shortdwarf.com
E talent@shortdwarf.com

Mannequin Model Agency & School
19148 Ten Mile Road
Eastpointe, MI 48021 USA
T 1 800 635 6335
F 1 810 775 4750

FACES FOR PLACES
22255 River Ridge Trail
Farmington Hills, MI 48335 USA
Contact: Judy Kulish, Owner
T 1 248 471 6611
F 1 248 471 6688

>>

MICHIGAN

Avante Model & Talent Agency & School
G-3490 Miller Road, Suite 15
Flint, MI 48507 USA
T 1 810 732 2233
F 1 810 732 1010

DIVINE MODELS & TALENT INC
7 Ionia South West, Suite 320
Grand Rapids, MI 49503 USA
Contact: Coleen Downey, Agency Director
T 1 616 774 9906
F 1 616 774 9907
E divineiwc@prodigy.net

PASTICHE MODELS & TALENT
1501 Lake Drive SE, Suite 292
Grand Rapids, MI 49506 USA
Contact: Bobby Haggard
T 1 616 451 2181
F 1 616 451 8417
E pastiche@iserv.net

Unique Models & Talent
4485 Plainfield North East, Suite 101C
Grand Rapids, MI 49525 USA
T 1 616 364 0959
F 1 616 364 5110

Adams' Pro Modeling School
2722 East Michigan Avenue, Suite 205
Lansing, MI 48912-4000 USA
T 1 517 482 4600
F 1 517 482 2185

CLASS MODELING & TALENT AGENCY
2722 East Michigan Avenue, Suite 205
Lansing, MI 48912-4000 USA
Contact: C.L. Adams, Owner
T 1 517 482 1833
F 1 517 482 2185

USA MODELS
107 Kalamazoo Street
Otsego, MI 49078 USA
Contact: Pam McQueer
T 1 616 692 3222
F 1 616 692 2806

THE CASTING GROUP
4830 N Parma Road
Parma, MI 49269 USA
Contact: Sue Kirchen, Owner
T 1 517 531 5250
F 1 517 531 4416

TRAQUE INT'L MODEL MANAGEMENT INC
316 1/2 S Main Street, Suite 201
Royal Oak, MI 48067 USA
Contact: Lynn Clark-Geiner, President
T 1 248 542 6355
F 1 248 542 6887
E traquemgmt@aol.com

John Robert Powers
26500 Northwestern, Suite 330
Southfield, MI 48076 USA
T 1 248 352 1234
F 1 248 352 2047

POWERS MODEL & TALENT AGENCY
26500 Northwestern, Suite 330
Southfield, MI 48076 USA
Contact: Judi March
T 1 248 352 2098
F 1 248 352 2047
W www.johnrobertpowers.net
E jrpdetroit@aol.com

John Casablancas/MTM
40840 Van Dyke Avenue
Sterling Heights, MI 48313 USA
T 1 810 795 9800
F 1 810 795 9834

AFFILIATED MODELS & TALENT GROUP
1680 Crooks Road
Troy, MI 48084 USA
Contact: Cathy Foreman
T 1 248 244 8770
F 1 248 244 0808
F 1 248 244 8731
E affilpromogh@aol.com

AERO MODEL MANAGEMENT
6230 Orchard Lake Road
W Bloomfield, MI 48322 USA
Contact: Sheryl Stokes
T 1 248 855 0251
F 1 248 855 3244

MODEL & TALENT AGENCIES

MINNESOTA

John Casablancas/MTM
8200 Humbolt Avenue S, Suite 101
Bloomington, MN 55431 USA
T 1 612 948 9000
F 1 612 948 1800

La Terese' Image Consulting & Modeling School/Agency
9811 54th Street
Clear Lake, MN 55319 USA
T 1 320 743 4200
F 1 320 743 3257

Minneapolis

ACADEMY OF FILM & TELEVISION
6651 Highway #7
Minneapolis, MN 55426 USA
T 1 612 915 9132
F 1 612 915 9181

CARYN INTERNATIONAL MODEL TRAINING CENTER
6651 Highway #7
Minneapolis, MN 55426 USA
Contact: Chuck Rosenberg
T 1 612 915 9132
F 1 612 915 9181

CARYN MODEL & TALENT AGENCY
100 N 6th Street, Suite 270B
Minneapolis, MN 55403 USA
Contact: Cindy Burke
SAG/AFTRA Franchised
T 1 612 349 3600
F 1 612 336 4445
W www.carynmodels.com

JOE KATZ MODELS
701 4th Avenue S, Suite 1700
Minneapolis, MN 55416 USA
Contact: Joe Katz
T 1 612 377 7630
F 1 612 337 3893

KIMBERLY FRANSON AGENCY
Hyatt Regency Complex,
1300 Nicollet Mall, Suite 220C
Minneapolis, MN 55403 USA
Contact: Kimberly Franson
T 1 612 386 4252
F 1 612 338 1411
W www.kimberlyfranson.com
E kfa@kimberlyfranson.com

MEREDITH MODEL & TALENT AGENCY
800 Washington Avenue North, Suite 511
Minneapolis, MN 55401 USA
Contact: Stacy Meredith
SAG/AFTRA Franchised
T 1 612 340 9555
T 1 973 812 0122 N.J. Office
F 1 612 340 9533

MOORE CREATIVE TALENT INC
1610 W Lake Street
Minneapolis, MN 55408 USA
Contact: Andrea Hjelm
SAG/AFTRA/AEA Franchised
T 1 612 827 3823
F 1 612 827 5345
E Available On Request

New Faces Models & Talent
6301 Wayzata Boulevard
Minneapolis, MN 55416 USA
T 1 612 544 8668
F 1 612 544 8932

Onyx Models Inc
2925 Dean Parkway, Suite 300
Minneapolis, MN 55416 USA
T 1 612 925 8343
F 1 612 922 4426

UNFORGETTABLE MODELS & TALENT AGENCY
4548 Abbott Avenue S
Minneapolis, MN 55410 USA
Contact: Easter Hailey, Director
T 1 952 842 8222
F 1 952 842 8288
E easterhailey@msn.com

WEHMANN MODELS & TALENT AGENCY
1128 Harmon Place, Suite 205
Minneapolis, MN 55403 USA
Contact: Susan Wehmann
AFTRA & SAG, Casting for Feature Films
T 1 612 333 6393
F 1 612 344 1444
W www.wehmann.com
E agents@wehmann.com

• • • • • • • • • • •

Kaye & Assoc Model & Talent Management
11 4th Street SE, Zumbro
Rochester, MN 55904 USA
T 1 507 286 1007
F 1 507 286 7492

Model Ink Avenue
1193 Earl Street
St Paul, MN 55106 USA
T 1 651 772 1670
F 1 651 772 1670

MTM AGENCY
1021 Bandana Boulevard
St Paul, MN 55108 USA
Contact: Robbyn Iverson, President
or Brian Nelson, Vice President
T 1 651 642 1222
F 1 651 642 1448
W www.johncasablancasmn-ny.com

MODEL & TALENT AGENCIES

MISSISSIPPI

Color Campus Model& Talent School & Agency
240 Eisenhower Drive, Bldg I-2
Biloxi, MS 39531-3648 USA
T 1 228 388 2465
F 1 228 388 2482

MODEL & TALENT AGENCIES

MISSOURI

Barbizon
7525 Forsyth Avenue
Clayton, MO 63105 USA
T 1 314 863 1141
F 1 734 758 0119

John Casablancas/MTM
1302 Virginia
Joplin, MO 64801 USA
T 1 501 444 7972
F 1 501 587 8555

Kansas City

EXPOSURE MODEL & TALENT AGENCY INC
215 West 18th Street
Kansas City, MO 64108 USA
Contact: Jennifer Mangan, Owner/Print Int'l Placement or Shawn Mullane, Owner/Broadcast
AFTRA Francised
T 1 816 842 4494
F 1 816 421 7575
W www.exposureinc.com
E exposure@kc.net

John Casablancas/MTM
221 E Gregory Boulevard
Kansas City, MO 64114 USA
T 1 816 361 2600

I & I Model Group LLC
1509 Westport Road
Kansas City, MO 64111 USA
T 1 816 410 9950
F 1 816 410 6944

MILLENNIUM MODEL MANAGEMENT
511 Delaware, Loft 100
Kansas City, MO 64105 USA
Contact: Terry Groman
T 1 816 474 8383
T 1 816 474 8384
W www.millennium-models.com
E tgroman@millennium-models.com
***See Ad Under Virginia Section.**

PATRICIA STEVENS MODEL AGENCY
2000 Baltimore Avenue
Kansas City, MO 64108-1914 USA
Contact: Melissa Stevens
Print • Fashion • TV • Conventions • Runway
T 1 816 221 1188
T 1 800 MODEL 01 Clients Only
F 1 816 221 2030
W www.patriciastevens.net
E psmodels@aol.com
***See Ad This Section.**

Talent Unlimited
4049 Pennsylvania Avenue
Kansas City, MO 64111 USA
T 1 816 561 9040
F 1 816 756 3950

• • • • • • • • • •

ALLURE MODELS
144 West Madison
Kirkwood, MO 63122 USA
Contact: Sue Wancel, Director
T 1 314 909 0666
F 1 314 909 0808

St Louis

CENTRO MODELS
1222 Lucas Avenue, Suite 300
St Louis, MO 63103 USA
Contact: Sharon Tucci, Owner
T 1 314 421 9400
F 1 314 421 9440
W www.centromodels.com
E talentplus-centro@talent-plus.com

CITY TALENT
2101 Locust, 2 West
St Louis, MO 63103 USA
Contact: June Evers, President
Lori Powell, Marketing Director
T 1 314 621 7200
F 1 314 621 1700
W www.city-talent.com
E info@city-talent.com

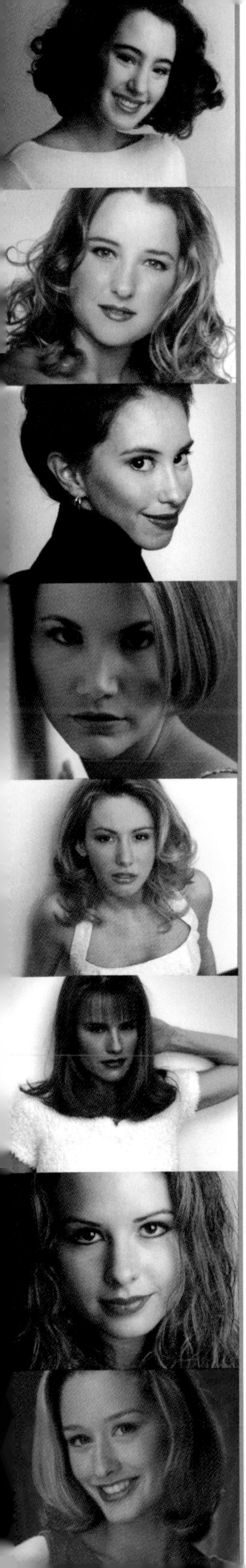

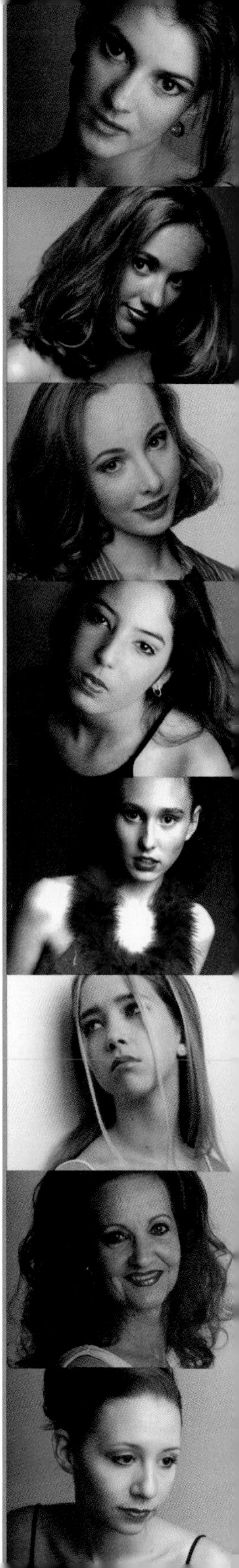

M INTERNATIONAL
1531 Washington Avenue, Suite 10-E
St Louis, MO 63103 USA
Contact: Barb Chan
T 1 314 436 0480
F 1 314 436 2992

PRIMA MODELS INC
522A S Hanley Road
St Louis, MO 63105 USA
Contact: Mark Dickmann
T 1 314 721 1235
F 1 314 721 3352
W www.primamodels.com
E PrimaModel@aol.com

TALENT PLUS INC
1222 Lucas Avenue, Suite 300
St Louis, MO 63103 USA
Contact: Sharon Tucci, Owner
T 1 314 421 9400
F 1 314 421 9440
W www.talent-plus.com
E talentplus-centro@talent-plus.com

THEE RASPBERRY COMPANY
1627 Washington Avenue, Suite 702
St Louis, MO 63103 USA
Contact: Robert Taliver Jr
T 1 314 436 8585
F 1 314 436 6512
W www.raspberrycompany.com
E models@raspberrycompany.com
E bobby.T@prodigy.net

• • • • • • • • • •

Professional Images Model & Talent
2571 W Landers Road
Springfield, MO 65714 USA
T 1 417 725 6580
F 1 417 725 6529

MODEL & TALENT AGENCIES

MONTANA

CREATIVE WORLD MODEL & TALENT
P.O. Box 50177
Billings, MT 59105-0177 USA
Contact: Lynette C. Michael, President
T 1 406 259 9540
F 1 406 245 7757
W www.creativeworldinc.com
E LCMichael@aol.com

MMTA • MONTANA'S MODEL & TALENT AGENCY
11332 Wineglass Lane
Livingston, MT 59047 USA
T 1 406 222 4699
F 1 406 222 4699

MODEL & TALENT AGENCIES

NEBRASKA

INTERNATIONAL SCHOOL OF MODELING
2806 S 110th Court
Omaha, NE 68144 USA
Contact: Traci Lenigan
T 1 402 399 8787
F 1 402 399 8789

NANCY BOUNDS MODEL & TALENT MANAGEMENT & SCHOOL
11915 Pierce Plaza
Omaha, NE 68144 USA
Contact: Mikeal Kay Loneman, Director
T 1 402 697 9292
F 1 402 697 9272
W www.nancyboundsmodels.com
E nancyboundsmodels@yahoo.com

Reel People Models & Talent
3036 North 102nd Street
Omaha, NE 68134 USA
T 1 402 734 2122
F 1 402 734 0909

EARTHBOUND ENTERTAINMENT, PROMOTIONS & TALENT
107 East E • P.O. Box 326
Wymore, NE 68466 USA
Contact: Billie Diekman, President
Nationwide Staffing for Event Marketing, Promotions, In-Store Demos, Casting & Production Management.
T 1 888 705 2008
F 1 402 645 8099
E earthbound@alltel.net

MODEL & TALENT AGENCIES

NEVADA

Las Vegas

ALAN WAXLER GROUP
3285 W Tompkins Avenue
Las Vegas, NV 89103 USA
Contact: Frances Carr, Director
T 1 702 792 8000
F 1 702 792 8011
W www.awaxgrp.com
E fran@awaxgrp.com

Baskow & Associates
2948 E Russell Road
Las Vegas, NV 89120 USA
T 1 702 733 7818
F 1 702 733 2052

EST MODELS & TALENT INC
4270 Cameron Street, Suite 6
Las Vegas, NV 89103 USA
Contact: Carrie Carter-Henderson
T 1 702 889 2900
F 1 702 889 2901
W www.bestmodelsandtalent.com
E chenderson@bestmodelsandtalent.com

LASSIC MODELS & TALENT
3305 Spring Mountain Road, Suite 12
Las Vegas, NV 89102 USA
Contact: Wendy Wenzel, President
T 1 702 367 1444
F 1 702 367 6457
E wwenzel997@aol.com

ENVY MODEL & TALENT
2121 Industrial Road, Loft 211
Las Vegas, NV 89102 USA
Contact: Daniel Mahan, Agency Director
T 1 702 878 7368
F 1 702 870 9750
W www.envymodels.com
E envymodels@mail.com

H.M.I. • HOLIDAY MODELS INC
900 East Desert Inn Road, Suite 101
Las Vegas, NV 89109-9300 USA
Contact: Kami Oisboid
T 1 702 735 7353
F 1 702 796 5676
W www.holidaymodels.com
E hmi@holidaymodels.com

JOHN ROBERT POWERS
3010 W Charleston, Suite 100
Las Vegas, NV 89102 USA
Contact: Kim Flowers, Executive Director
T 1 702 878 7300
F 1 702 880 0871
W www.lasvegastalent.com
E KFStyles@aol.com

LENZ AGENCY PEOPLE WITH TALENT
1591 E Desert Inn Road
Las Vegas, NV 89109 USA
Contact: Richard Weber
T 1 702 733 6888
F 1 702 731 2008
W www.lenztalent.com
E richardweber@lenztalent.com

MCCARTY TALENT INC
4220 S Maryland Parkway, Suite B317
Las Vegas , NV 89119 USA
Contact: W. Cody Garden
T 1 702 944 4440
F 1 702 944 4441
W www.mccartytalent.com
E agent@mccarty.com

Supreme Agency
4180 S Sandhill Road, Suite B8
Las Vegas, NV 89121 USA
T 1 702 433 3393
F 1 702 458 0442

• • • • • • • • • • •

Creative Model Management
1029 Riverside Drive
Reno, NV 89503-5430 USA
T 1 775 348 2001
F 1 775 348 7785

John Robert Powers
9490 Gateway Drive, Suite 110
Reno, NV 89511 USA
T 1 775 851 2062
F 1 775 851 2065

MODEL & TALENT AGENCIES

NEW HAMPSHIRE

CINDERELLA MODELING AGENCY
9 Brook Street
Manchester, NH 03104 USA
Contact: Suzette Paradis
Serving the Boston & New England Market
T 1 603 627 4125 NH Office
F 1 603 669 5785 NH Fax
T 1 781 324 7590 MA Office
F 1 781 324 4875 MA Fax
W www.cinderellamodelsne.com
E cindmod@msn.com

NEW ENGLAND MODELS GROUP INC
250 Commercial Street, Suite 2022
Manchester, NH 03101 USA
Contact: Kathleen Longsderff
T 1 603 624 0555
F 1 603 624 4188
W www.nemg.com
E nemodels@nemg.com

Savage Pageantry International
22 S Broadway
Salem, NH 03079 USA
T 1 603 894 9734

MODEL & TALENT AGENCIES

NEW JERSEY

McCullough Models & Talent
8 S Hanover Avenue
Atlantic City, NJ 08402 USA
T 1 609 822 2222
F 1 609 823 3333

CLASSIC MODEL AND TALENT MANAGEMENT
87 South Finley Avenue
Basking Ridge, NJ 07920 USA
Contact: Kathy Nedved
T 1 908 766 6663
F 1 908 766 3053
W www.rivint.com/classic
E classic@rivint.com
***See Ad This Section.**

KD Casting
383 N Kings Highway, Suite 5B
Cherry Hill, NJ 08034 USA
T 1 609 482 9113
F 1 609 667 2341

MODELS ON THE MOVE MODEL & TALENT AGENCY
1200 Route 70, Barclay Towers, Suite 6,
Cherry Hill, NJ 08034 USA
Contact: Lucy King
AFTRA & SAG Francised
T 1 856 667 1060
F 1 856 667 8363

ZUR INC PROMOTIONAL/TALENT AGENCY
329 Myrtle Street • P.O. Box 42
Cliffwood, NJ 07721 USA
Models, Singers, Actors & Dancers...Worldwide
Established 1960
T 1 732 566 9282
F 1 732 566 2850
W www.zur-inc.com
E talent@zur-inc.com

Nationwide Talent Inc
P.O. Box 2423
Clifton, NJ 07015 USA
T 1 973 340 3600
F 1 973 340 8323

BEAUTI-FIT TALENT AGENCY
P.O. Box 559
Closter, NJ 07624 USA
Contact: Kenny Kassel
Specializing in Athletic / Fit Models.
T 1 212 459 4472
T 1 201 767 1444
C 1 201 280 5484
F 1 201 767 1011
W www.beautifit.com
***See Ad Under NYC Model Agencies.**

Kids.com
186 Fairfield Road
Fairfield, NJ 07004 USA
T 1 973 575 7300
F 1 973 575 2610

BARBIZON AGENCY OF PARAMUS
440 Route 17 North, Suite 4
Hasbrouck Heights, NJ 07604 USA
Contact: Ron or Jackie Gerbino
T 1 201 727 1034
F 1 201 727 1039
E barbizonnj@aol.com

CLERI MODELS
402 Main Street, Suite 300
Metuchen, NJ 08840 USA
Contact: Frank Cleri
Representing the All-American to International looks for Fashion, Editorial, Catalogue, Commercial Print, TV & Film
T 1 732 632 9544
T 1 212 721 6900 New York
T 1 732 632 9545 Model Mgmt
F 1 732 321 1046
***See Ad Under NYC Model Agencies.**

AXIS MODELS & TALENT INC
46 Church Street
Montclair, NJ 07042 USA
Contact: Sharon Norrell / Dwight Brown
T 1 973 783 4900
F 1 973 783 8081

Barbizon
70 Park Street
Montclair, NJ 07042 USA
T 1 973 783 4030
F 1 973 783 0368

Total Talent Management
40 Enclosure
Nutley, NJ 07110 USA
T 1 973 661 4923
F 1 973 661 1185

MODEL TEAM MODEL MANAGEMENT LLC
55 Central Avenue
Ocean Grove, NJ 07756 USA
Contact: John Merriman
Representing Men, Women & Children (Ages 5 & up)
Featured On "Good Day, New York,"
European T.V. and ABC-TV!
T 1 732 988 3648
F 1 732 988 9262
***See Ad Under NYC & New Jersey Sections.**

Barbizon
80 Broad Street
Red Bank, NJ 07701 USA
T 1 732 842 6161

COVER GIRL STUDIO MODEL MANAGEMENT
630 Kinderkamack Road
River Edge, NJ 07661 USA
Contact: Cliff Adam
T 1 201 261 2042
F 1 201 261 2047
W www.covergirlmodelmgt.com

NATORI'S CLUB
71 South Orange Avenue, #385
South Orange, NJ 07079 USA
Contact: Alnisia Cruz, Booking Director
Childrens Agency for Print, Catalog & Television.
T 1 973 762 5091
F 1 973 762 5032
W www.natori-club.com
E acruz@natori-club.com

MEREDITH MODEL & TALENT AGENCY
10 Furler Street
Totowa, NJ 07512 USA
Contact: Joyce Meredith
SAG/AFTRA Franchised
T 1 973 812 0122
T 1 612 340 9555 MN Office
F 1 973 812 0141

BARBIZON
P.O. Box 3909
Trenton, NJ 08629 USA
Contact: Dawn Fitch, Director
T 1 609 586 3310
E barbizonsilkmodels@aol.com

Blanche Zeller Productions
27 Waldeck Court
West Orange, NJ 07052 USA
T 1 973 324 1534
F 1 973 324 1537

≫

MODEL & TALENT AGENCIES

NEW MEXICO

Albuquerque

THE EATON AGENCY
3636 High Street NE
Albuquerque, NM 87107 USA
Contact: Abigail Eaton
T 1 505 344 3149
F 1 505 344 3018
W www.eatonagency.com
E eatonagency@earthlink.net

John Robert Powers
2021 San Mateo NE
Albuquerque, NM 87110 USA
T 1 505 266 5677
F 1 505 266 6829

Phoenix Agency
8809 Washington Street, Suit 100
Albuquerque, NM 87113 USA
T 1 505 797 1940
F 1 505 797 1905

Red Nations Native American Model & Talent Agency
2930 Monroe NE
Albuquerque, NM 87110 USA
T 1 505 837 1585

MODEL & TALENT AGENCIES

NEW YORK STATE

Barbizon
1991 Central Avenue
Albany, NY 12205 USA
T 1 518 456 6713
F 1 518 456 6715

Conwell Career Centre
137 Summer Street
Buffalo, NY 14222-2205 USA
T 1 716 884 0763
F 1 716 882 8931

LAUNCH MT
5600 Strickler Road
Clarence, NY 14031 USA
T 1 716 741 3033
F 1 716 741 8245

Nexus Personal Management
P.O. Box 614
Fairport, NY 14450 USA
T 1 716 425 1377
F 1 716 425 1362

JOHN CASABLANCAS / MTM AGENCY
69-02 Austin Street, Suite 210
Forest Hills, NY 11375 USA
Contact: Robbyn Iverson, President
or Brian Nelson, Vice President
T 1 718 997 0718
F 1 718 997 0728
W www.johncasablancasmn-ny.com

Christina Models
55 S Bergen Place, Suite 4E
Freeport, NY 11520 USA
T 1 516 868 5932

New Faces Model Management
25 Woodbury Road
Hicksville, NY 11801 USA
T 1 516 822 4208
F 1 516 938 1725

Vanique Models
25 Woodbury Road
Hicksville, NY 11801 USA
T 1 516 938 1701
F 1 516 938 1725

JENNIFER MODELS INC AGENCY
P.O. Box 20170
Huntington Station, NY 11746 USA
T 1 631 385 4924
F 1 631 385 4925
W www.jennifermodels.com
E staff@jennifermodels.com

M Model Management
350 Route 110
Huntington Station, NY 11746 USA
T 1 516 425 7235
F 1 516 271 0387

HOLLYWOOD IMAGE MODEL & TALENT AGENCY
247 W Montauk Highway
Lindenhurst, NY 11757 USA
Contact: Rich Herbeck, President
T 1 631 226 0356
F 1 631 226 0373
W www.hollywoodimageagency.com

CLAIRE MODEL & TALENT MANAGEMENT
168 West Park Avenue
Long Beach, NY 11561 USA
Contact: Clarice
T 1 516 897 3703
F 1 516 889 4889
E Clairemdl@aol.com

MARY THERESE FRIEL LLC
1251 Pittsford Mendon Road
Mendon, NY 14506 USA
Contact: Mary Therese Friel & Kent Friel
T 1 716 624 5510
F 1 716 582 1268
W www.mtfmodels.com
E youcanbe@frontiernet.net

Elaine Gordon Model Management
2942 Harbor Road
Merrick, NY 11566 USA
T 1 212 936 1001
F 1 516 623 8863

Joanne's Modeling
69 Ironwood Road
New Hartford, NY 13413 USA
T 1 315 797 6424

MODEL & TALENT AGENCIES

NEW YORK CITY

Abrams Artists Agency
275 Seventh Avenue, 26th Floor
New York, NY 10001 USA
T 1 646 486 4600
F 1 646 486 0100

ADONIS MODEL MANAGEMENT
451 Greenwich Street, Suite 504
New York, NY 10013 USA
Contact: Anne Marie Principe
T 1 212 807 0055
F 1 212 206 1608

APM MODEL MANAGEMENT INC
20 W 20th Street, 6th Floor
New York, NY 10010 USA
Contact: Penny Basch / Louise Roberts
T 1 212 352 9230
F 1 212 633 8741
W www.apmmodelmanagement.com
E apmmodel@aol.com

>>

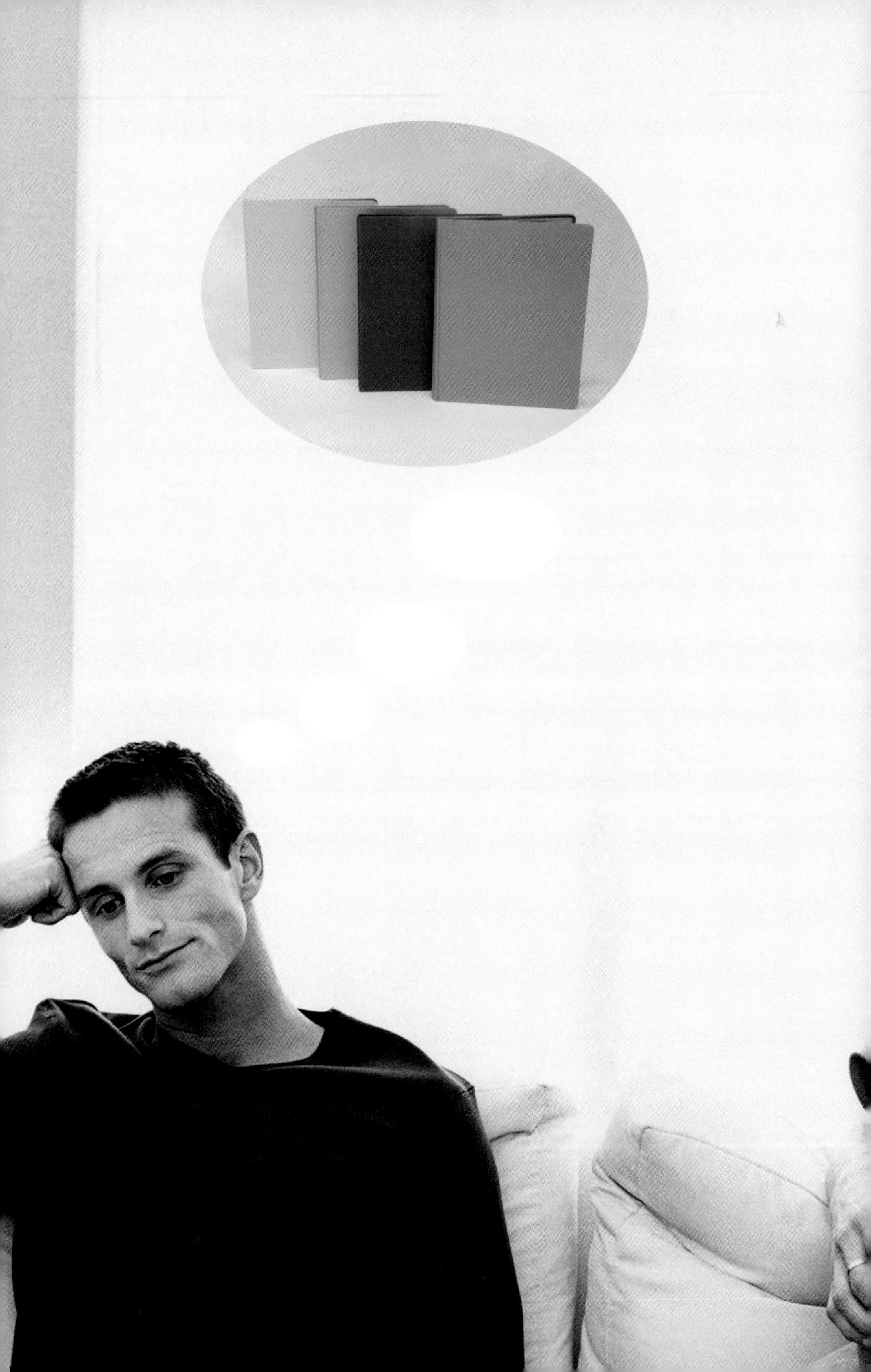

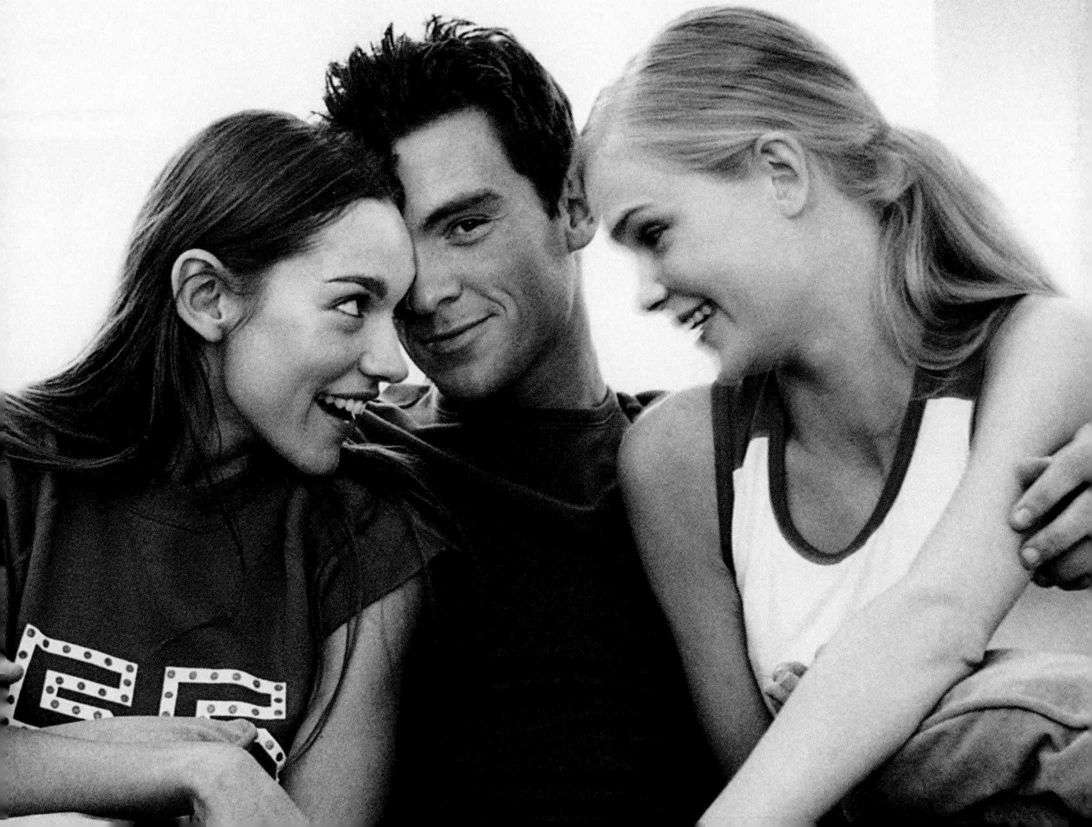

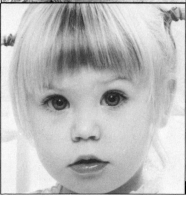

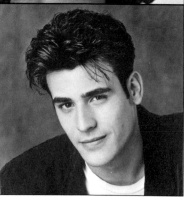

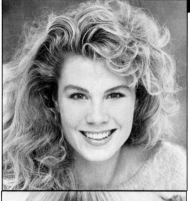

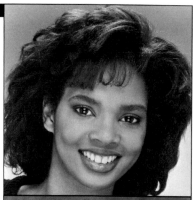

BARBIZON AGENCY
15 Penn Plaza
New York, NY 10001 USA
Promotions, Trade Shows, Hostesses; Est. 1939
T 1 212 239 1110
T 1 718 230 0550
F 1 212 967 4256
***See Ad This Section.**

Boss Models
1 Gansevoort Street
New York, NY 10014 USA
T 1 212 242 2444
F 1 212 633 6127

Clear Model Management
625 Broadway, 6th Floor
New York, NY 10012 USA
T 1 212 353 5058
F 1 212 777 4174

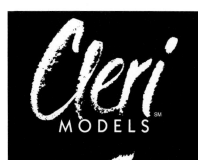

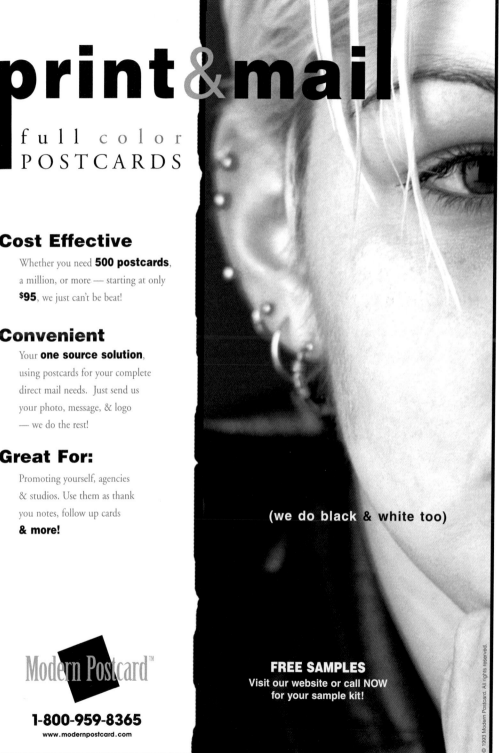

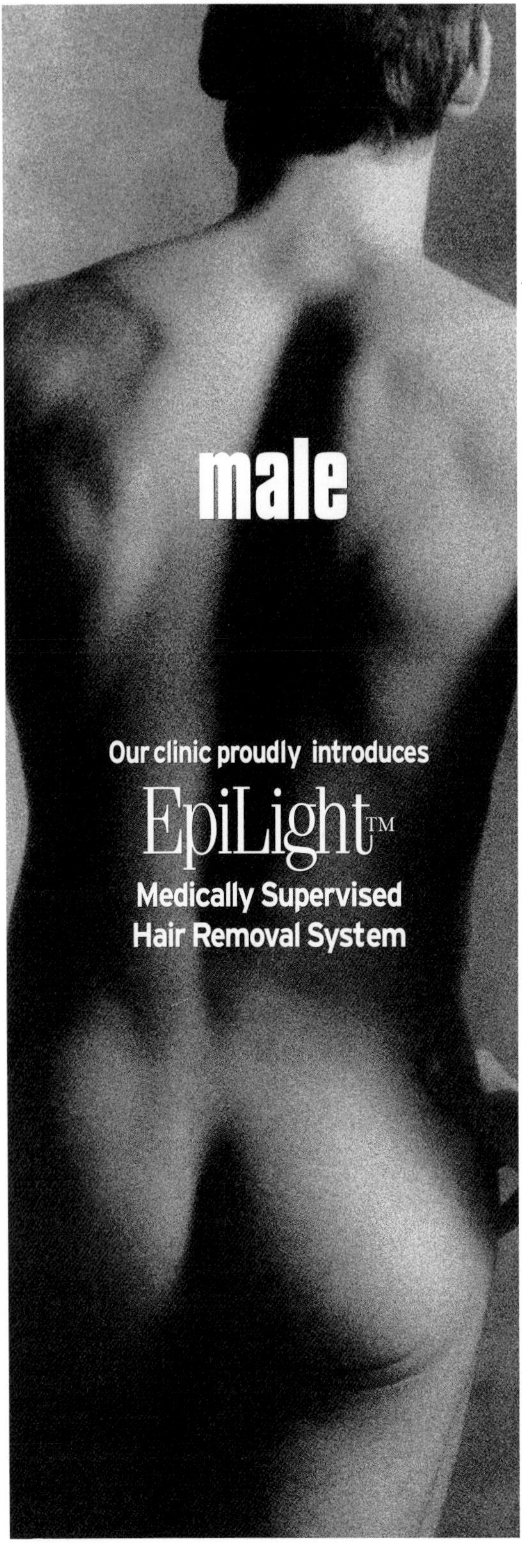
male
Our clinic proudly introduces
EpiLight™
Medically Supervised
Hair Removal System

Click Models
129 W 27th Street
New York, NY 10001 USA
T 1 212 206 1616
F 1 212 206 6228

COMPANY MANAGEMENT
270 Lafayette Street, Suite 1400
New York, NY 10012 USA
Michael Flutie, President
T 1 212 226 9190 General Info
F 1 212 226 9791
E CompanyNYC@aol.com

CUNNINGHAM, ESCOTT & DIPENE
257 Park Avenue South, Suite 900
New York, NY 10010 USA
Contact: Sharon Reich, Print Division
T 1 212 477 3838
F 1 212 673 2359
W www.cedtalent.com
E info@cedtalent.com

CURVES AT THE LYONS GROUP
505 Eighth Avenue, Floor 12 A, Studio 1
New York, NY 10008 USA
Contact: Kathy Backer
T 1 212 239 3539
F 1 212 239 4221
W www.lyonsgroupny.com
E kathybacker@lyonsgroupny.com

DIVA MODEL MANAGEMENT
451 Greenwich Street, Suite 504
New York, NY 10013 USA
Contact: Anne Marie Principe
T 1 212 807 0055
F 1 212 206 1608

ELEMENT 119
304 Park Ave South, Suite 606
New York, NY 10010 USA
T 1 212 460 8544
F 1 212 460 8543

Elite Model Management
111 E 22nd Street
New York, NY 10010 USA
T 1 212 529 9700
F 1 212 475 0572

Elite Runway
111 E 22nd Street
New York, NY 10010 USA
T 1 212 995 7317
F 1 212 475 0572

FFT / FUNNYFACE TODAY INC
17 W 17th Street, 8th Floor
New York, NY 10011 USA
Contact: Jane Blum
T 1 212 686 4343
F 1 212 689 8619
W www.fftmodels.com
E fft@fftmodels.com
***See Ad This Section.**

FLAUNT MODEL MANAGEMENT INC
114 E 32nd Street, Suite 501
New York, NY 10016 USA
Contact: Gene Roseman, President
Representing Men and Women, SAG/AFTRA Francised
T 1 212 679 9011
F 1 212 679 0938
E flauntmodels@earthlink.com

FORCE INTERNATIONAL
350 Fifth Avenue, 71st Floor
New York, NY 10118 USA
Contact: Rudy DeVaughn, Director
T 1 212 736 9042
F 1 212 736 6086
E rdevaughn@forceintl.com

FORD MODELS
142 Greene Street, 4th Floor
New York, NY 10012 USA
T 1 212 219 6500
F 1 212 966 1531
W www.fordmodels.com
***See Ad This Section.**

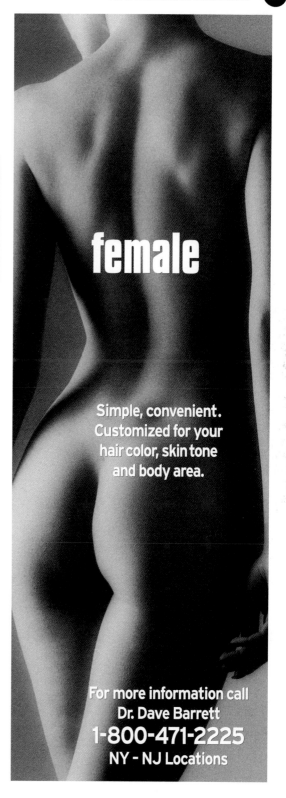

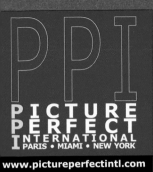

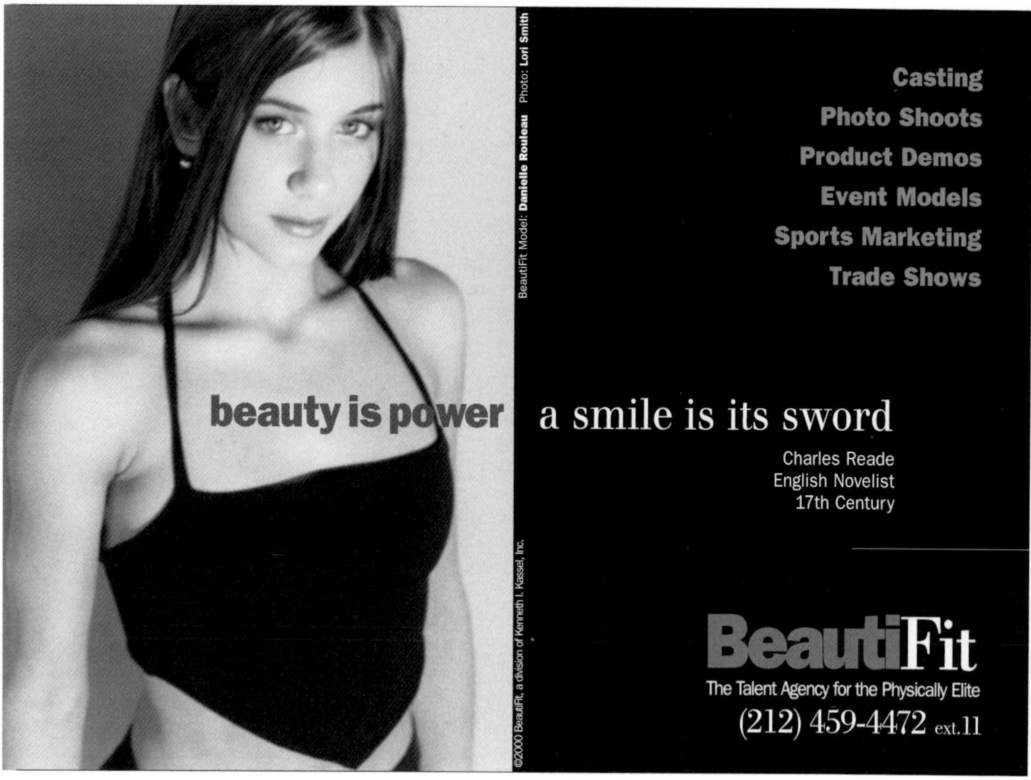

FOSTER FELL
234 Fifth Avenue, Suite 406
New York, NY 10001 USA
T 1 212 532 2227
F 1 212 532 2272
E JeremyFY@aol.com

GILLA ROOS LTD
16 W 22nd Street, 3rd Floor
New York, NY 10010 USA
Contact: David Roos, President
T 1 212 727 7820
F 1 212 727 7833
W www.gillaroos.com
E talent@gillaroos.com

Gotham Model Management
357 West Broadway, 3rd Floor
New York, NY 10013 USA
T 1 212 431 0100
F 1 212 431 6258

GRACE DEL MARCO
350 Fifth Avenue, Suite 3110
New York, NY 10118 USA
Contact: Dee Simmons-Edelstein, Director
T 1 212 629 6404
F 1 212 629 6403
W www.gracedelmarco.com
***See Ad This Section**

GRAMERCY MODELS INC
234 Fifth Avenue, Suite 506
New York, NY 10001 USA
Contact: Vicki Sasso, President
T 1 212 481 1227
F 1 212 779 3493
W www.gramercymodelsny.com
E models928@aol.com

HILLARY BECKFORD MODEL MANAGEMENT / MAD
15 Penn Plaza, Room 34, Office Level 2
New York, NY 10001 USA
Contact: Hillary Beckford, President
T 1 212 563 3313
T 1 212 871 5521
F 1 212 631 0196
E missbeckford@aol.com

ID MEN
137 Varick Street
New York, NY 10013 USA
T 1 212 334 4333
F 1 212 334 4999
W www.idmodels.com
E men@idmodels.com

ID MODEL MANAGEMENT
137 Varick Street
New York, NY 10013 USA
T 1 212 941 5858 Women
F 1 212 941 5776
W www.idmodels.com
E info@idmodels.com

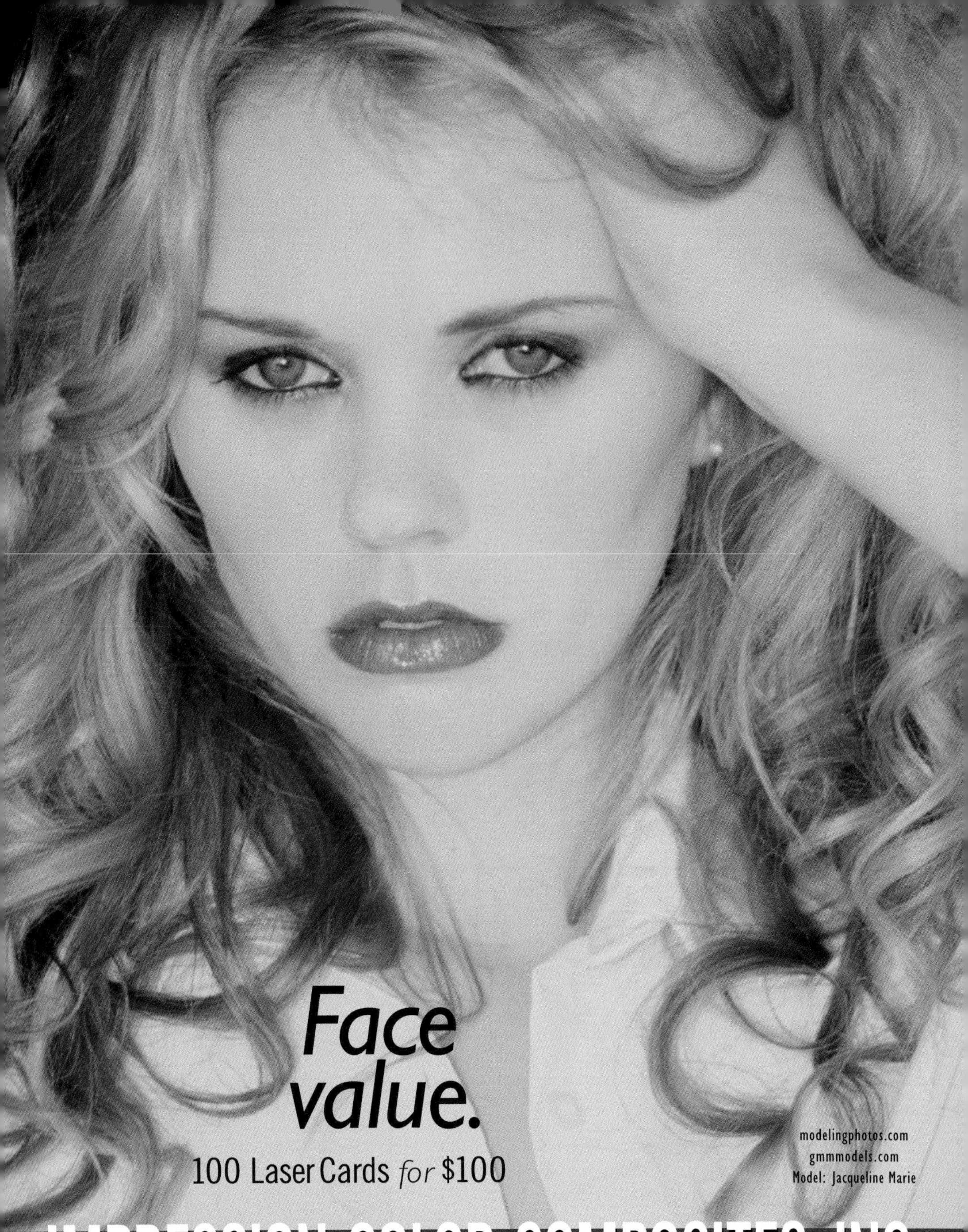
Face value.
100 Laser Cards for $100
modelingphotos.com
gmmmodels.com
Model: Jacqueline Marie

NYC MODELING AGENCIES

Ikon New York
140 E 22nd Street, 2nd Floor
New York, NY 10011 USA
T 1 212 691 2363
F 1 212 691 3622

IMAGES MANAGEMENT • WOMEN
30 E 20th Street
New York, NY 10003 USA
T 1 212 228 0300
F 1 212 228 0438

IMG MODELS
304 Park Ave South, Penthouse North
New York, NY 10010 USA
Contact: Jan Planit, Director
T 1 212 253 8882
F 1 212 253 8883
W www.imgworld.com
E modelinfo@imgworld.com
***See Ad This Section.**

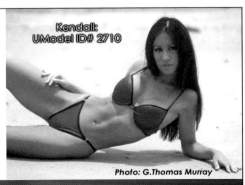

JAN ALPERT MODEL MANAGEMENT
333 E 55th Street, Suite 7G
New York, NY 10022 USA
By Appointment Only.
T 1 212 223 4238
F 1 212 223 9244

JOHN ROBERT POWERS
90 West Street, Suite 1612
New York, NY 10006 USA
Contact: Giampiero Paoletti, President
T 1 212 267 8900
F 1 212 267 2364
W www.johnrobertpowers.net
E jrpnewyork@aol.com

KARIN MODELS • NEW YORK
6 West 14th Street, 3rd Floor
New York, NY 10011 USA
Contact: Scott Lipp, President
T 1 212 334 6400
T 1 212 226 4100 Women
F 1 212 226 4060 Women Fax
T 1 212 996 4200 Men
F 1 212 966 3733 Men Fax
T 1 212 966 7991 Artists
F 1 212 431 5293 Artists Fax
New 646 Numbers take effect 2.20.2001
T 1 646 638 3330 Women
F 1 646 638 2123 Women Fax
T 1 646 638 3331 Men
F 1 646 638 1909 Men Fax
T 1 646 638 2413 Artists
F 1 646 638 2130 Artists Fax
T 1 646 638 3722 Executive & Accounting
F 1 646 638 3738 Executive & Accounting Fax
W www.karinmodels.com

LITTLE MACS/MCDR TEENS
156 Fifth Avenue, Suite 222
New York, NY 10010 USA
Contact: Angela Buie
Commercial Print • Fashion Print
T 1 212 627 3100
F 1 212 627 7293
E ab@mcdrmodels.com
*See Ad This Section.

THE LYONS GROUP
505 Eighth Avenue, Floor 12 A, Studio 1
New York, NY 10008 USA
Contact: Mike Lyons
T 1 212 239 3539
F 1 212 239 4221
W www.lyonsgroupny.com
E Lyonsgrpny@aol.com

M MODEL MANAGEMENT
352 Seventh Avenue, Suite 431
New York, NY 10001 USA
T 1 212 631 7551
F 1 212 631 7574

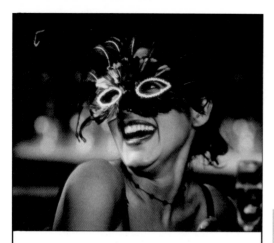

MODELS FOR CHRIST

PURPOSE

Models for Christ seeks to encourage and strengthen the spiritual growth of all those interested within the fashion business.

Since 1984 Models for Christ has been a lighthouse within the darkness of the fashion industry.

Models, photographers, agents, designers and others involved in the fashion business volunteer their time and energy to maintain this non-profit organization.

We provide helpful resources for spiritual growth, sponsor outreach projects, hold regular Bible studies, and connect fashion professionals with fellowship in Paris, Milan, Tokyo and other major fashion capitals.

REACHING OUT TO THOSE WHO ARE LESS FORTUNATE.

Children undergoing life saving cancer treatment appreciate a smile from anyone willing to take the time to care. At right, Jim gets an unusual make-up job at our MFC St. Patrick's Day party, while face painting with a child at the Ronald McDonald House in NYC.

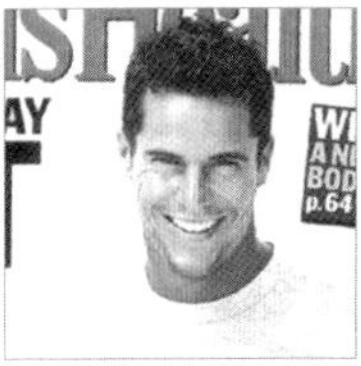

BRADLY @ NEXT

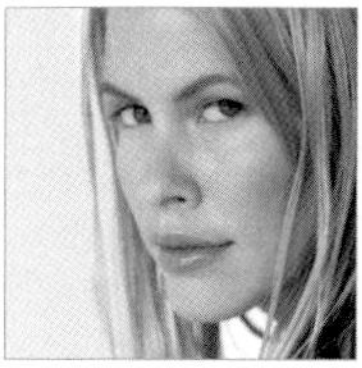

CHRISTINA @ CLICK

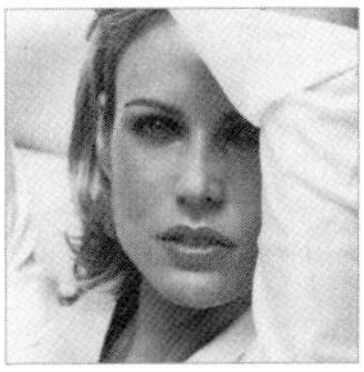

DAWN @ ELITE

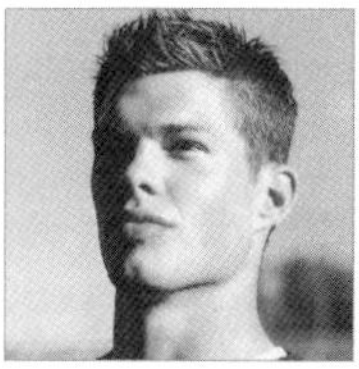

WILL @ FORD

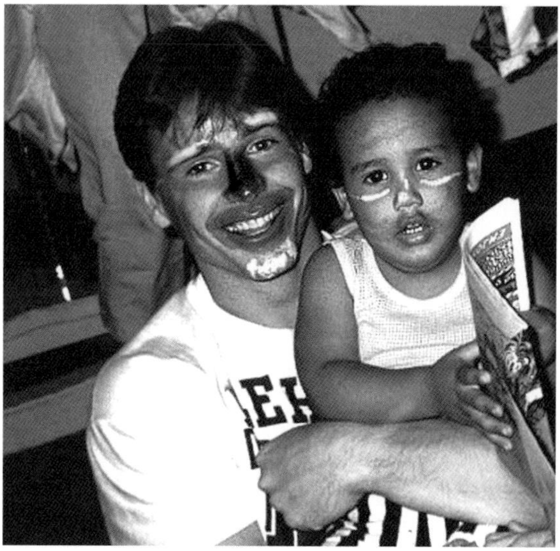

VISIT WWW.**MODELSFORCHRIST.COM** TO LEARN MORE ABOUT THIS PROJECT AND 17 OTHER MFC COMMUNITY SERVICE PROJECT IDEAS YOU CAN TRY IN YOUR TOWN. JUST CLICK ON THE BUTTON "GIVING BACK".

M·F·C·

Light in the darkness

MODELS FOR CHRIST, 54 WEST 39TH ST. 3RD FLOOR, NEW YORK, NY 10018
PH: 212.780.4881 / E-MAIL: AGENTS@MODELSFORCHRIST.COM / WWW.MODELSFORCHRIST.COM

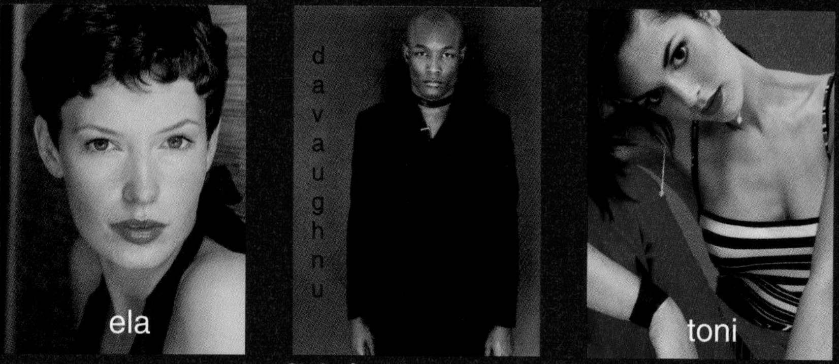

MADISON MODELS
84 Wooster Street, 4th Floor
New York, NY 10012 USA
Contact: Eduard Pesch
T 1 212 941 5577
F 1 212 941 5559
W www.madisonmodels.com
E info@madisonmodels.com

MAJOR MODEL MANAGEMENT
381 Park Avenue South, Suite 1501
New York, NY 10016 USA
T 1 212 685 1200
F 1 212 683 5200
E majormodelmgmt@aol.com

Marilyn Inc
300 Park Avenue South
New York, NY 10010 USA
T 1 212 260 6500
F 1 212 260 0821

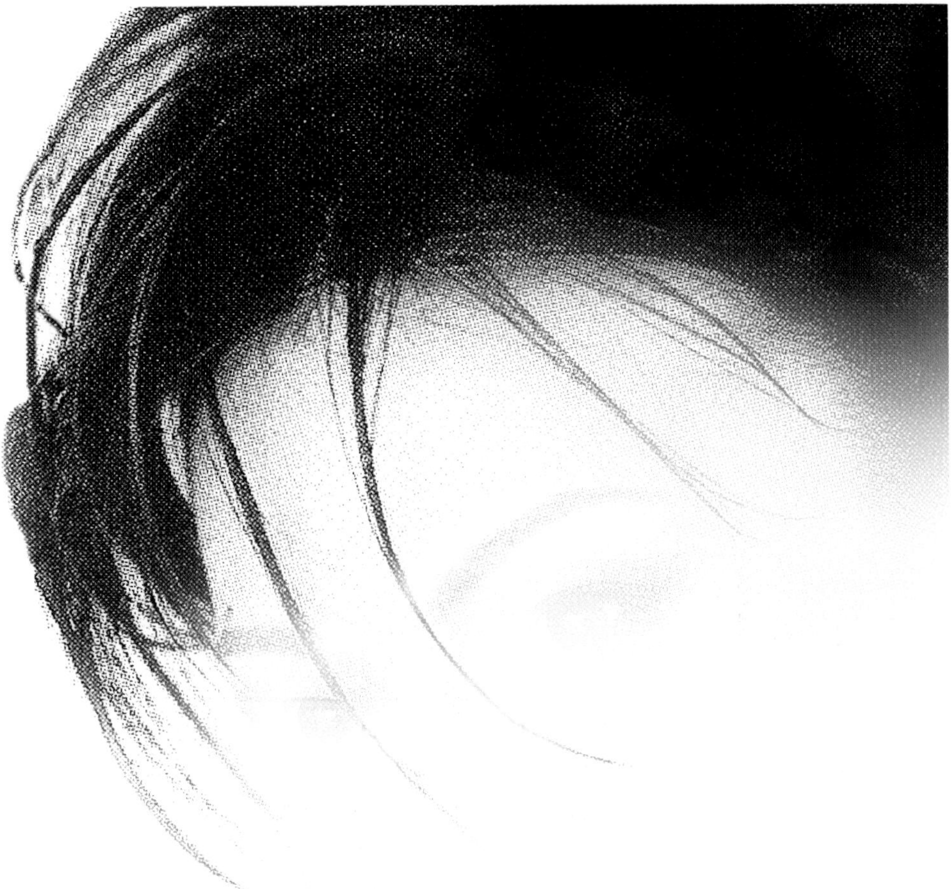

MAXX MEN
30 E 20th Street
New York, NY 10003 USA
T 1 212 228 0278
F 1 212 228 0438

McDONALD/RICHARDS
156 Fifth Avenue, Suite 222
New York, NY 10010 USA
Contact: Gary Bertalovitz, President
Commercial Print • Catalog
T 1 212 627 3100
F 1 212 627 7293
W www.mcdonaldrichardsmodels.com
E gjb@mcdrmodels.com
*See Ad This Section.

NYC MODELING AGENCIES

MCDR NYC MEN
156 Fifth Avenue, Suite 222
New York, NY 10010 USA
Contact: Vonetta Lynn
Fashion • Catalog • Editorial
Showroom • Fit • Body
T 1 212 352 2617
F 1 212 627 7293
W www.mcdonaldrichardsmodels.com
E men@mcdrmodels.com
***See Ad This Section.**

MCDR NYC WOMEN
156 Fifth Avenue, Suite 222
New York, NY 10010 USA
Contact: Marielle Cardone / Alvin de La Pena
Fashion • Catalog • Editorial
Showroom • Runway • Fit
T 1 212 352 2617
F 1 212 627 7293
E women2@mcdrmodels.com
***See Ad This Section.**

Mega Management
59 E Franklin Street, Suite B9
New York, NY 10013 USA
T 1 212 334 5800
F 1 212 334 9164

Metropolitan Models
220 Fifth Avenue, Suite 800
New York, NY 10001 USA
T 1 212 481 0500
F 1 212 481 2525

MODEL & TALENT MANAGEMENT
415 Seventh Avenue
New York, NY 10001 USA
Print, Fashion, Acting & TV Commercials
T 1 212 239 1110
F 1 212 967 4256
***See Ad This Section.**

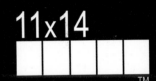

NEW YORK MODEL MANAGEMENT
596 Broadway, Suite 701
New York, NY 10012 USA

T	1 212 539 1700
F	1 212 539 1775
W	www.newyorkmodels.com
E	women@newyorkmodels.com
E	men@newyorkmodels.com
E	runway@newyorkmodels.com

*See Ad This Section.

NEXT MANAGEMENT • NEW YORK
23 Watts Street
New York, NY 10013 USA

T	1 212 925 5100	Main
T	1 212 925 3900	Women
T	1 212 925 5300	Women
T	1 212 334 3337	Men
F	1 212 925 5948	Men Fax
T	1 212 226 2225	New Faces
T	1 212 925 5996	Artists New York
F	1 212 941 8483	Artists Fax
F	1 212 925 5931	
W	www.nextmodelmanagement.com	

*See Ad This Section.

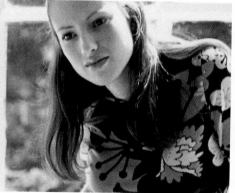

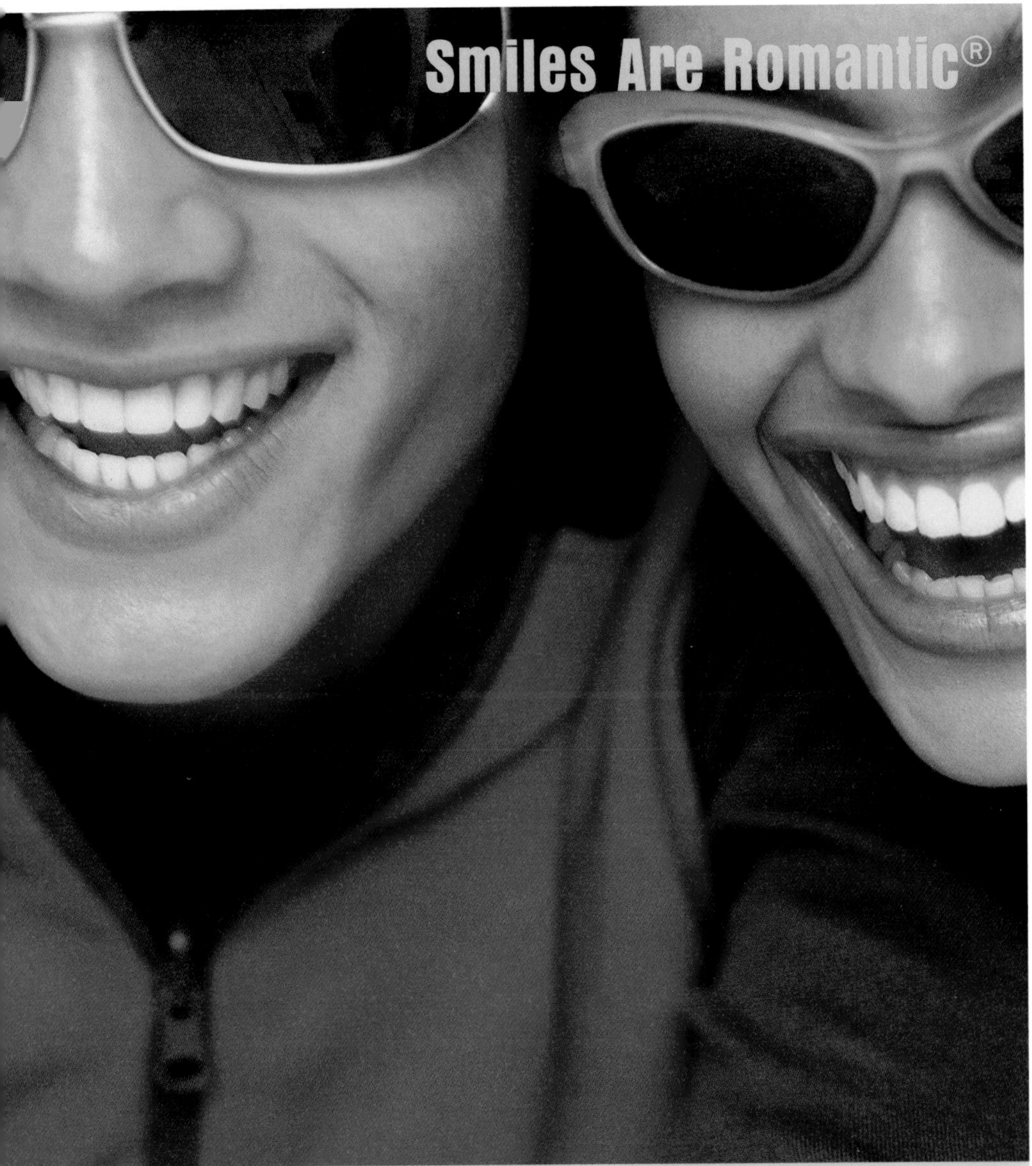
Smiles Are Romantic®

NMK • NEEDHAM METZ KOWALL
19 W 21st Street, Suite 401
New York, NY 10010 USA
Contact: Ken Metz / Debbi Kowall
T 1 212 741 7000
F 1 212 741 7007
W www.nmkmodels.com
E nmkmod@aol.com

OHM Management
1133 Broadway, Suite 910
New York, NY 10001 USA
T 212 989 6395
F 212 989 3860

PARTS MODELS
P.O. Box 7529, FDR Station
New York, NY 10150 USA
Contact: Danielle Korwin, Owner
T 1 212 744 6123
F 1 212 396 3014
W www.partmodels.com
E info@partmodels.com

PAULINE'S MODEL MANAGEMENT
379 West Broadway, Suite 502
New York, NY 10012 USA
Contact: Pauline Bernachez, President
T 1 212 941 6000
F 1 212 274 0434
W www.paulinesonline.com
E info@paulinesonline.com

PEOPLE MODEL & TALENT MANAGEMENT
137 Varick Street
New York, NY 10013 USA
T 1 212 941 9800
F 1 212 941 5776
W www.peopleagency.com
E info@peopleagency.com

PERFORMANCE EVENT MARKETING INC
1133 Broadway, Suite 1403
New York, NY 10010 USA
Contact: Michael Glickman, President
Specializing in staffing local and national promotions with models & actors. New talent please mail head shots and resumes (no calls).
T 1 212 206 6956
F 1 212 229 1774
W www.pemonline.com
E michaelg@pemonline.com

Q MODEL MANAGEMENT
180 Varick Street, 13th Floor
New York, NY 10014 USA
Contact: Gwenn Saiman or Jeffrey Kolsrud
T 1 212 807 6777 Women
T 1 212 807 6111 Men
F 1 212 807 8999
W www.qmodels.com
E nyc@qmodels.com
*See Ad This Section.

R & L MODEL MANAGEMENT
203 W 23rd Street, Suite 400
New York, NY 10011 USA
T 1 212 935 2300
F 1 646 638 3368

REQUEST MODEL MANAGEMENT
119 W 22nd Street, 2nd Floor
New York, NY 10011 USA
T 1 212 924 4241
F 1 212 463 7274
E requestmodels@juno.com

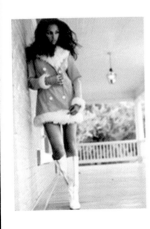

T MANAGEMENT
91 Fifth Avenue, 3rd Floor
New York, NY 10003 USA
Contact: Annie Veltri, President
T 1 212 924 0990
F 1 212 645 4940
E tmanagement@tmgmt.com

Thompson Model & Talent Management
50 West 34th Street, Suite 6C6,
New York, NY 10001 USA
T 1 212 947 6711
F 1 212 947 6732

TOMORROW TALENT
915 Broadway, Suite 1306
New York, NY 10011 USA
Contact: Deniece
T 1 212 777 8811
F 1 212 777 6360
E Modelclub1@AOL.com

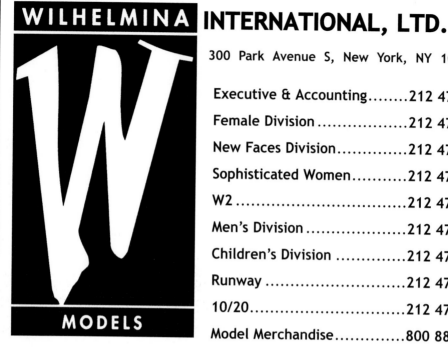

WILHELMINA INTERNATIONAL LTD
300 Park Avenue South, 2nd Floor
New York, NY 10010 USA
T 1 212 473 4610 Female Division
T 1 212 473 2198 Men's Division
T 1 212 473 3651 New Faces Division
T 1 212 473 1253 Children's Division
T 1 212 473 0700 Executive & Accounting
T 1 212 473 4138 Runway
T 1 212 473 3952 Sophisticated Women
T 1 212 473 4884 10/20
T 1 212 473 1613 W2
T 1 800 889 6633 Model Merchandise
F 1 212 473 3223
***See Ad This Section.**

Women Model Management
199 Lafayette Street, 7th Floor
New York, NY 10012 USA
T 1 212 334 7480
F 1 212 334 7492

ZOLI MANAGEMENT INC
3 West 18th Street, 5th Floor
New York, NY 10011-4699 USA
T 1 212 242 1500 Information
T 1 212 242 5959 Women
T 1 212 242 6060 Men
F 1 212 242 7505

MODELING AGENCIES, CHILDREN

NEW YORK CITY

Ford/Children
142 Greene Street, 4th Floor
New York, NY 10012 USA
T 1 212 219 6150
F 1 212 219 6156

GENERATION MODEL MGMT INC
20 West 20th Street, Suite 1008
New York, NY 10011 USA
Contact: Patti Fleischer
T 1 212 727 7219
F 1 212 727 7147

LITTLE MACS/MCDR TEENS
156 Fifth Avenue, Suite 222
New York, NY 10010 USA
Contact: Angela Buie
Commercial Print • Fashion Print
T 1 212 627 3100
F 1 212 627 7293
E ab@mcdrmodels.com
***See Ad This Section.**

PRODUCT MODEL MANAGEMENT INC
240 W 35th Street, Suite 1001
New York, NY 10001 USA
Contact: Alyson, Michael or Charles
T 1 212 563 6444
F 1 212 465 1967
E product@banet.net

WILHELMINA CREATIVE MANAGEMENT
300 Park Avenue South, 2nd Floor
New York, NY 10010 USA
Infants to 12 years old
T 1 212 473 1253
T 1 212 979 9797 TV
T 1 212 271 1601 TV
F 1 212 473 3223
***See Ad This Section.**

PERSONAL MANAGERS

NEW YORK

Adele's Kids • Adults Mgmt
33 Rupert Avenue
Staten Island, NY 10314 USA
T 1 718 494 5000
F 1 718 494 2933

Bieller Management
445 W 45th Street
New York, NY 10036 USA
T 1 800 451 5813
F 1 800 236 7071

Cuzzins Management
250 W 57th Street
New York, NY 10107 USA
T 1 212 765 6559

Debbie's Kids
14 Tamara Lane
Cornwalle, NY 12518 USA
T 1 914 534 3485

Dee Mura Enterprises Inc
269 West Shore drive
Massapequa, NY 11758 USA
T 1 516 795 1616

Flutie Entertainment Corp
270 Lafayette Street, Suite 1400
New York, NY 10012 USA
T 1 212 226 7001

Fox Entertainment Co Inc
1650 Broadway, Suite 503
New York, NY 10019 USA
T 1 212 582 9072

Fresh Faces Management
2911 Carnation Avenue
Baldwin, NY 11510-4402 USA
T 1 516 223 0034
F 1 516 379 0353

Goldstar Talent Management Inc
850 Seventh Avenue, Suite 904
New York, NY 10019 USA
T 1 212 315 4429
F 1 212 315 4574

Green Key Management
251 W 89th Street
New York, NY 10024
T 1 212 874 7373

Harry Bellovin
410 E 64th Street
New York, NY 10021 USA
T 1 212 752 5181

Jennifer Lambert
1600 Broadway, Suite 1001
New York, NY 10019 USA
T 1 212 315 0665

Joseph Rapp Ents
1650 Broadway
New York, NY 10019 USA
T 1 212 265 3366

Joyce Chase Management
2 Fifth Avenue
New York, NY 10011 USA
T 1 212 473 1234

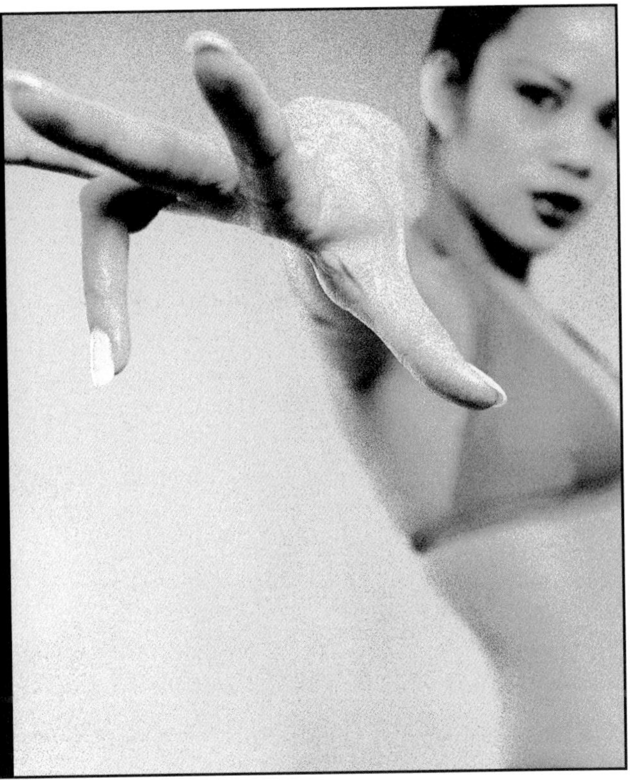

Knowles Management
234 E 52nd Street, Suite B
New York, NY 10022 USA
T 1 212 750 2330

Landside Management
155 E 76th Street, Suite 12A
New York, NY 10021 USA
T 1 212 585 4230

Lloyd Kolmer Ents
65 W 55th Street
New York, NY 10019 USA
T 1 212 582 4735

Michael Katz Management
P.O. Box 1925, Cathedral Station
New York, NY 10025 USA
T 1 212 316 2492

Michele Donay Talent Mgmt
76 W 86th
New York, NY 10024-3607 USA
T 1 212 769 0924

Monica Management
1050 Fifth Avenue
New York, NY 10028 USA
T 1 212 860 7101

Nani-Saperstein Management
1600 Broadway, Suite 605
New York, NY 10019 USA
T 1 212 582 7690

Podesoir International Management
211 W 56th Street, Suite 4J
New York, NY 10019 USA
T 1 212 767 0520

Rosella Olson Management
319 W 105th Street
New York, NY 10025 USA
T 1 212 864 0336

Sandi Merle
101 W 57th Street
New York, NY 10019 USA
T 1 212 489 1578

SUZELLE ENTERPRISES
100 W 57th Street, Suite 15E,
New York, NY 10019 USA
Contact: Suzanne Schachter
T 1 212 397 2047
F 1 212 397 2032
W www.avotaynu.com/suzelle

>>

NYC PERSONAL MANAGERS

Terrific Talent
419 Park Avenue S, Suite 1009
New York, NY 10016 USA
T 1 212 689 2800
F 1 212 481 1000

Think Tank Talent
389 Fifth Avenue, Suite 1010
New York, NY 10016 USA
T 1 914 237 5834

Top Drawer Entertainment
108-39 Union Turnpike
Forest Hills, NY 11375 USA
T 1 718 896 4001

Val Irving
30 Park Avenue
New York, NY 10016 USA
T 1 212 685 5496

Vic Ramos Management
49 W 9th Street
New York, NY 10011 USA
T 1 212 473 2610

Whatley Management & Production Company
315 E 57th Street
New York, NY 10022 USA
T 1 212 308 9682

Young Talent Inc
P.O. Box 792
Hartsdale,, NY 10530 USA
T 1 914 948 4744

TALENT AGENCIES

NEW YORK

Abrams Artists Agency
275 Seventh Avenue, 26th Floor
New York, NY 10001 USA
T 1 646 486 4600
F 1 646 486 0100

Agency For Performing Arts
888 Seventh Avenue
New York, NY 10106 USA
T 1 212 582 1500
F 1 212 245 1647

Agents For The Arts
203 W 23rd Street
New York, NY 10011 USA
T 1 212 229 2562
F 1 212 463 9313

Amererican International Talent Agency
303 W 42nd Street, Suite 608
New York, NY 10036 USA
T 1 212 245 8888
F 1 212 245 8926

Andreadis Talent Agency
119 W 57th Street
New York, NY 10019 USA
T 1 212 315 0303
F 1 212 315 0311

Archer King Ltd
244 W 54th Street, 12th Floor
New York, NY 10019 USA
T 1 212 765 3103
F 1 212 765 3107

Artists Group East
1650 Broadway, Suite 610
New York, NY 10019 USA
T 1 212 586 1452
F 1 212 586 0037

Associated Booking
1995 Broadway, Suite 501
New York, NY 10023 USA
T 1 212 874 2400
F 1 212 769 3649

Babs Zimmerman Productions
305 E 86th Street, Suite 17 FW
New York, NY 10028 USA
T 1 212 348 7203

Baby Wranglers Casting Inc
689 Fort Washington Avenue, Suite 1AA
New York, NY 10040 USA
T 1 212 568 1200
F 1 212 568 1200

Barry, Haft, Brown Artists Agency
165 W 46th Street
New York, NY 10036 USA
T 1 212 869 9310
F 1 212 398 1268

Bauman, Redanty & Shaul
250 W 57th Street
New York, NY 10019 USA
T 1 212 757 0098
F 1 212 489 8531

Berman, Boals & Flynn Inc
208 W 30th Street, Suite 401
New York, NY 10012 USA
T 1 212 868 1068

The Bethel Agency
311 W 43rd Street, Suite 602
New York, NY 10036 USA
T 1 212 664 0455

Beverly Anderson
1501 Broadway, Suite 2008
New York, NY 10036 USA
T 1 212 944 7773

Bret Adams
448 W 44th Street
New York, NY 10036 USA
T 1 212 765 5630
F 1 212 265 2212

Bruce Levy Agency
311 W 43rd Street, Suite 602
New York, NY 10036 USA
T 1 212 262 6845
F 1 212 262 6846

Buchwald & Associates Inc
10 E 44th Street
New York, NY 10017 USA
T 1 212 867 1200
F 1 212 867 2434

Carry Company
49 W 46th Street, 4th Floor
New York, NY 10036 USA
T 1 212 768 2793
F 1 212 768 2713

Carson-Adler Agency
250 W 57th Street, Suite 808
New York, NY 10107 USA
T 1 212 307 1882
F 1 212 541 7008

Carson Organization Ltd
240 W 44th Street, Penthouse
New York, NY 10036 USA
T 1 212 221 1517

Coleman-Rosenburg
155 E 55th Street, Suite 5D
New York, NY 10022 USA
T 1 212 838 0734
F 1 212 838 0774

CUNNINGHAM, ESCOTT & DIPENE
257 Park Avenue South, Suite 900/950
New York, NY 10010 USA
Voice Over: Sharon Bierut
On Camera: Ken Slevin
Children: Halle Madia
T 1 212 477 1666
T 1 212 477 6622 Children
F 1 212 979 2011
W www.cedtalent.com
E info@cedtalent.com

Dorothy Palmer Talent Agency
235 W 56th Street, Suite 24K
New York, NY 10019 USA
T 1 212 765 4280
F 1 212 765 4280

Douglas, Gorman, Rothacker & Wilhelm Inc
1501 Broadway, Suite 703
New York, NY 10036 USA
T 1 212 382 2000
F 1 212 397 0307

Dulcina Eisen Associates
154 E 61st Street
New York, NY 10021 USA
T 1 212 355 6617
F 1 212 355 6723

Duva-Flack Associates
200 W 57th Street, Suite 1008
New York, NY 10019 USA
T 1 212 957 9600
F 1 212 957 9606

Edie Robb Talent Works
301 W 53rd Street
New York, NY 10019 USA
T 1 212 245 3250
F 1 212 245 2853

EWCR & Associates
311 W 43rd Street
New York, NY 10036 USA
T 1 212 586 9110
F 1 212 586 8019

Fifi Oscard Agency Inc
24 W 40th Street, 17th Floor
New York, NY 10018 USA
T 1 212 764 1100
F 1 212 840 5019

Frontier Booking International Inc
1560 Broadway, Suite 1110
New York, NY 10036 USA
T 1 212 221 0220

Funnyface Today Inc
17 W 17th Street, 8th Floor
New York, NY 10011 USA
T 1 212 686 4343
F 1 212 685 6861

Gage Group Inc
315 W 57th Street, Suite 4H
New York, NY 10019 USA
T 1 212 541 5250
F 1 212 956 7466

>>

NYC TALENT AGENCIES

Gersh Agency
130 W 42nd Street, Suite 2400
New York, NY 10036 USA
T 1 212 997 1818
F 1 212 391 8459

Ginger Dicce Talent Agency
1650 Broadway, Suite 714
New York, NY 10019 USA
T 1 212 974 7455

Hanns Wolters Agency
10 W 37th Street
New York, NY 10018 USA
T 1 212 714 0100
F 1 212 643 1412

Harry Packwood Talent Ltd
250 W 57th Street, Suite 2012
New York, NY 10107 USA
T 1 212 586 8900
F 1 212 265 9122

HWA Talent Representatives
220 E 23rd Street, Suite 400
New York, NY 10010 USA
T 1 212 889 0800
F 1 212 889 1643

Henderson/Hogan Agency Inc
850 Seventh Avenue, Suite 1003
New York, NY 10019 USA
T 1 212 765 5190
F 1 212 586 2855

Ingber & Associates
274 Madison Avenue, Suite 1104
New York, NY 10016 USA
T 1 212 889 9450
F 1 212 779 0490

Innovative Artists
141 Fifth Avenue, 3rd Floor
New York, NY 10010 USA
T 1 212 253 6900
F 1 212 253 1198

International Creative Management
40 W 57th Street
New York, NY 10019 USA
T 1 212 556 5600
F 1 212 556 5665

Jerry Kahn Inc
853 Seventh Avenue, Suite 7C
New York, NY 10019 USA
T 1 212 245 7317
F 1 212 582 9898

J Mitchell Management
440 Park Avenue, S 11th Floor
New York, NY 10016 USA
T 1 212 679 3550

Jordan, Gill & Dornbaum
156 Fifth Avenue, Suite 711
New York, NY 10010-7002 USA
T 1 212 463 8455
F 1 212 691 6111

KMA Agency
11 Broadway, Suite 1101
New York, NY 10004 USA
T 1 212 581 4610
F 1 212 422 1283

Kerin-Goldberg & Associates
155 E 55th Street, Suite 5D
New York, NY 10022 USA
T 1 212 838 7373
F 1 212 838 0774

Krasny Office Inc
1501 Broadway, Room 1303
New York, NY 10036 USA
T 1 212 730 8160
F 1 212 768 9379

Lally Talent Agency
630 Ninth Avenue, Suite 800
New York, NY 10036 USA
T 1 212 974 8718

LBH Associates Inc
1 Lincoln Plaza
New York, NY 10023 USA
T 1 212 501 8936
F 1 212 877 8647

Lionel Larner Ltd
119 W 57th Street, Suite 1412
New York, NY 10019-2401 USA
T 1 212 246 3105
F 1 212 956 2851

Michael Hartig Agency
156 Fifth Avenue
New York, NY 10010 USA
T 1 212 929 1772
F 1 212 929 1266

Norman Reich Agency
1650 Broadway, Suite 303
New York, NY 10019 USA
T 1 212 399 2881
F 1 212 581 4457

ouvelle Talent Management Inc
453 W 17th Street, 3rd Floor
New York, NY 10011 USA
T 1 212 645 0940
F 1 212 242 6466

mnipop Inc Talent Agency
55 W Old Country Road
Hicksville, NY 11801 USA
T 1 516 937 6011
F 1 516 937 6209

ppenheim-Christie Associates
13 E 37th Street, 7th Floor
New York, NY 10016 USA
T 1 212 213 4330
F 1 212 213 4754

aradigm
200 W 57th Street, Suite 900
New York, NY 10019 USA
T 1 212 246 1030
F 1 212 246 1521

Peggy Hadley Ents
250 W 57th Street
New York, NY 10107 USA
T 1 212 246 2166
F 1 212 756 2418

Peter Beilin Agency
230 Park Avenue, Suite 200
New York, NY 10169 USA
T 1 212 949 9119

Peter Strain & Associates Inc
1501 Broadway, Suite 2900
New York, NY 10036 USA
T 1 212 391 0380
F 1 212 391 1405

Professional Artists Unltd
321 W 44th Street, Suite 605
New York, NY 10036 USA
T 1 212 247 8770
F 1 212 977 5686

RADIOACTIVE TALENT INC
350 Third Avenue, Suite 400
New York, NY 10010 USA
Do not Phone or visit; mail all inquiries.

Rapp Enterprises Inc
1650 Broadway, Suite 1410
New York, NY 10019 USA
T 1 212 247 6646

Richard Astor Agency
250 W 57th Street, Suite 2014
New York, NY 10019 USA
T 1 212 581 1970
F 1 212 581 1980

Sames & Rollnick Associates
250 W 57th Street, Suite 703
New York, NY 10107-0703 USA
T 1 212 315 4434
F 1 212 582 0122

Schuller Talent/NY Kids
276 Fifth Avenue, Suite 207
New York, NY 10001 USA
T 1 212 532 6005
F 1 212 779 3479

Silver, Massetti & Szatmary
145 W 45th Street, Suite 1204
New York, NY 10036 USA
T 1 212 391 4545
F 1 212 354 4941

Spotlight Entertainment
322 Bowling Green
New York, NY 10274 USA
T 1 212 675 4297
F 1 212 675 8622

Talent Reps Inc
20 E 53rd Street
New York, NY 10022 USA
T 1 212 752 1835
F 1 212 752 7558

Tantleef Office
375 Greenwich Street, Suite 700
New York, NY 10013 USA
T 1 212 941 3939
F 1 212 941 3948

TRH Talent Agency
600 Madison Avenue, 23rd Floor
New York, NY 10022 USA
T 1 212 371 7500
F 1 212 371 7509

Universal Attractions
225 W 57th Street
New York, NY 10019 USA
T 1 212 582 7575
F 1 212 333 4508

Waters & Nicolosi
1501 Broadway, Suite 1305
New York, NY 10036 USA
T 1 212 302 8787
F 1 212 382 1019

>>

NYC TALENT AGENCIES

William Morris Agency
1325 Sixth Avenue
New York, NY 10019 USA
T 1 212 586 5100
F 1 212 246 3583

William Schill Agency
250 W 57th Street, Suite 2402
New York, NY 10107 USA
T 1 212 315 5919
F 1 212 397 7366

Writers & Artists Agency
19 W 44th Street
New York, NY 10036 USA
T 1 212 391 1112
F 1 212 398 9877

VARIETY/CIRCUS AGENCIES

NEW YORK

MICHAEL BONGAR ENTERTAINMENT
553 8th Street, Suite 2H
Brooklyn, NY 11215 USA
Contact: Michael Bongar
T 1 718 832 8268
F 1 718 832 8273
W www.michaelbongar.com

MODEL & TALENT AGENCIES

NEW YORK STATE CONTINUED

Magnificent Models Inc
120-53 Springfield Boulevard
Queens, NY 11411 USA
T 1 718 978 6020

US TALENT MANAGEMENT INC
250 N Goodman Street, Studio 3-6
Rochester, NY 14607 USA
Contact: Billy Powell, President
or Jennifer Boothby, Agency Director
T 1 716 244 0592
F 1 716 244 4324
W www.ustalent.com
E mail@ustalent.com

Personal Best
3653 Harlem Road
Snyder, NY 14215 USA
T 1 716 839 9012
F 1 716 831 3872

Barbizon Modeling School
190 East Post Road
White Plains, NY 10601 USA
T 1 914 428 2030
F 1 914 428 3367

TANNEN'S TALENT & MODEL MANAGEMENT
77 Tarrytown Road
White Plains, NY 10607 USA
Contact: Lynne Tannen
T 1 914 946 0900
F 1 914 946 1547
Babies-Children-Teens-Adults

UMODELS.COM
2 William Street, Suite 202
White Plains, NY 10601 USA
Contact: Michael D. Schneider, President
T 1 800 4 UMODELS
F 1 914 682 3683
W www.umodels.com
E mail@umodels.com
***See Ad Under NYC Model Agencies.**

Tomorrow Talent
20 crossways Park N
Woodbury, NY 11796 USA
T 1 212 777 8811

MODEL & TALENT AGENCIES

NORTH CAROLINA

TALENT TREK • ASHEVILLE
PMB 356, 825-C Merrimon Avenue
Asheville, NC 28804 USA
Contact: Juanell Walker / Charlotte Dennison
T 1 828 251 0173
F 1 865 977 9200
W www.talentrek.com
E talentrek@mindspring.com

Charlotte

CAROLINA TALENT
1201 S Graham Street, Suite 201
Charlotte, NC 28203 USA
Contact: Randy Motsinger, President
T 1 704 332 3218
F 1 704 343 2593
W www.carolinatalentinc.com
E carolinatalent@hotmail.com

ICE MODEL & TALENT MANAGEMENT
McMullen Creek Market,
8318 Pineville-Matthews Road, Suite 265
Charlotte, NC 28226 USA
Contact: Pamela Jones
T 1 704 543 4120
F 1 704 542 4744
W www.icemodels.com
E ice@icemodels.com

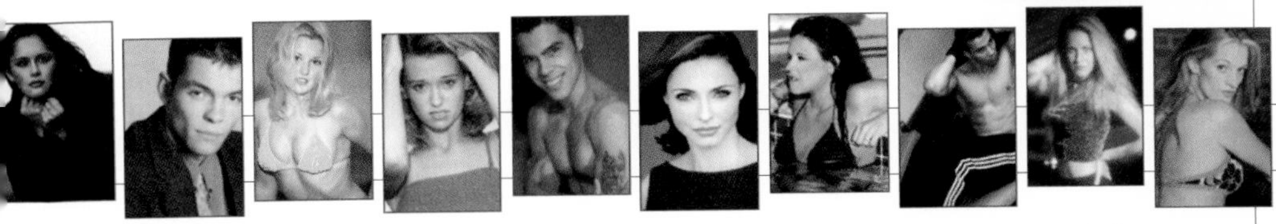

John Casablancas/MTM
810 Tyvola Road, Suite 100
Charlotte, NC 28217 USA
T 1 704 523 6966
F 1 704 523 3091

John Robert Powers
915 E 4th Street, Suite B
Charlotte, NC 28204 USA
T 1 704 358 9010
F 1 704 358 6711

JTA Talent Inc
820 East Boulevard
Charlotte, NC 28203 USA
T 1 704 377 5987
F 1 704 377 5854

Libby Stone Modeling School & Agency
1819 Charlotte Drive
Charlotte, NC 28203 USA
T 1 704 377 9299
F 1 704 358 8109

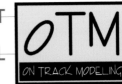

Model Select International
4919 Albemarie Road, Suite 203
Charlotte, NC 28205
T 704 536 7760
F 704 536 3155

ON TRACK MODELING INC
5500 Executive Center Drive, Suite 223
Charlotte, NC 28212 USA
Contact: RD Ecksmith
T 1 704 532 6577
F 1 704 532 6220
***See Ad This Section.**

SASS MODELING & TALENT AGENCY
5501 Executive Center Drive, Suite 232
Charlotte, NC 28212 USA
Contact: Terri Alexander
T 1 704 567 9393
F 1 704 567 1811
E sassagency@alltel.net

• • • • • • • • • • •

FACE NATIONAL MODELS & TALENT
19501 West Catawba Avenue, Suite 10
Cornelius, NC 28031 USA
Contact: Jennifer Gill
T 1 704 895 8123
F 1 704 987 0475

SILHOUETTES INC
P.O. Box 1079
Elon College, NC 27244 USA
Contact: Lori Wright
T 1 336 226 7450
F 1 336 570 0766
W www.silhouettesinc.com
E silhouettes@mindspring.com

Roland's School & Modeling Agency
310 Hope Mills Road
Fayetteville, NC 28304 USA
T 1 910 424 0409

Suzanne's Modeling Studio
2502 E Ash Street
Goldsboro, NC 27534 USA
T 1 919 734 7038

Touch of Class
P.O. Box 942
Goldsboro, NC 27530 USA
T 1 919 736 7665
F 1 919 736 8700

DIRECTIONS USA
3717C Market Street
Greensboro, NC 27403 USA
Contact: Jean Catlett
Specializing in Fashion Print, Commercials, Film, Hair and Makeup Artists & Stylists.
T 1 336 292 2800
F 1 336 292 2855
W www.directionsusa.com
E newfaces@directionsusa.com

MARILYN'S MODEL & TALENT AGENCY
60l Norwalk Street
Greensboro, NC 27407 USA
Promotions: Scottie Seaver
Print/New Faces: Freda Snyder
TV/Film: Kathy Moore
T 1 336 292 5950
F 1 336 294 9178
W www.marilyn-s.com
E models@marilyn-s.com
E scottie@marilyn-s.com
*See Ad This Section

THE TALENT CONNECTION
338 N Elm Street, Suite 204
Greensboro, NC 27401 USA
Contact: Anne Swindell
T 1 336 274 2499
F 1 336 274 9202
E talcongso@aol.com

THE BROCK AGENCY
329 13th Avenue NW
Hickory, NC 28601 USA
Contact: Beverly J Brock, President
T 1 828 322 8553
F 1 828 322 3224
W www.thebrockagency.com
E talent@twave.net

Creative Connections
607 Main Avenue SW
Hickory, NC 28602-2601 USA
T 1 828 327 3349
F 1 828 397 7114

JOAN BAKER STUDIO
403 Country Club Acres
Kings Mountain, NC 28086 USA
Contact: Joan Baker
T 1 704 739 6868
F 1 704 739 6866

CB GROUP TALENT MANAGEMENT
1253 Colony Drive
New Bern, NC 28562 USA
Contact: Connie Beddow
T 1 252 638 6912
F 1 252 638 6946
W www.cbgroup.com
E cbtalent@aol.com

Barbizon
4109 Wake Forest Road, Suite 400
Raleigh, NC 27609 USA
T 1 919 876 8201
F 1 919 876 6475

John Casablancas/MTM
4326 Bland Road
Raleigh, NC 27609 USA
T 1 919 878 0911
F 1 919 954 9008

JOHN ROBERT POWERS
4600 Marriott Drive, Suite 300
Raleigh, NC 27612 USA
Contact: Anila Wali, Executive Director
T 1 919 786 9898
F 1 919 786 9022
W www.johnrobertpowers.com
E jrpraleighnc@aol.com

DELIA MODEL & TALENT MANAGEMENT INC
1519 N 23rd Street, Suite 203
Wilmington, NC 28405 USA
Contact: Delia Harper
T 1 910 343 1753
T 1 910 343 0690
F 1 910 343 9473
E DMMMDLS@aol.com

Maultsby Talent-The Talent Source Training Center
112 N Cardinal Drive, Cardinal Place, Suite 106
Wilmington, NC 28405 USA
T 1 910 313 0922
F 1 910 313 0922

Capri & Associates
895 Peters Creek Parkway, Suite 204
Winston-Salem, NC 27103 USA
T 1 336 725 4102
F 1 336 773 1168

Vision Quest Models Agency
5020 Hutchins Street
Winston-Salem, NC 27106 USA
T 1 336 924 5076
F 1 336 924 3966

MODEL & TALENT AGENCIES
NORTH DAKOTA

Academie Agencie
220 Broadway, Suite B
Fargo, ND 58102 USA
T 1 701 235 8132
F 1 701 235 0027

MODEL & TALENT AGENCIES
OHIO

Barbizon
3296 W Market Street
Akron, OH 44333 USA
T 1 330 867 4110
F 1 330 867 0214

PRO-MODEL MANAGEMENT
3296 W Market Street
Akron, OH 44333 USA
Contact: Katie Logan
T 1 330 867 4125
F 1 330 867 0214
W www.promodelmgmt.com
E katie@promodelmgmt.com

Barbizon
750 W Resource Drive, Suite 20
Brooklyn Heights, OH 44131-1836 USA
T 1 216 351 8100
F 1 216 642 5449

Cincinnati

ASHLEY TALENT AGENCY
10948 Reading Road, Suite 310 & 311
Cincinnati OH 45241 USA
Contact: Pat Webster
T 1 513 554 4836
F 1 513 554 4838

CAM TALENT
1150 W 8th Street, Suite 262
Cincinnati OH 45203 USA
Contact: Carrie Ellen Zappa
T 1 513 421 1795
F 1 513 421 0122
W www.camtalent.com
E camtalent@aol.com

Cincinnati Model Agency
6047 Montgomery Road
Cincinnati, OH 45213 USA
T 1 513 351 2700
F 1 513 351 2702

>>

HEYMAN TALENT
3308 Brotherton Road
Cincinnati, OH 45209 USA
Contact: Anne James, Print Director
SAG/AFTRA Francised
T 1 513 533 3113
T 1 800 851 7077 Toll Free
F 1 513 533 3135
W www.heymantalent.com
E heyman@one.net

NEW VIEW MANAGEMENT GROUP
10680 McSwain Drive
Cincinnati, OH 45241 USA
Contact: Joe Guerrera, President
T 1 513 733 4444
F 1 513 733 0054
W www.nvmodels.com
E joe@nvmodels.com

WINGS MODEL AGENCY
906 Main Street, Suite 207
Cincinnati, OH 45202 USA
Contact: Jake Lang, Owner/Director
T 1 513 929 9464
F 1 513 929 9444
W www.wingsmodels.com

Cleveland

D'AVILA MODEL & TALENT MANAGEMENT
5840 Ridge Road
Cleveland, OH 44129 USA
Contact: Barbara D'Avila
T 1 440 843 7200
F 1 440 843 8084

FORD CLEVELAND
1300 E 9th Street, Suite 1640
Cleveland, OH 44114 USA
T 1 216 522 1300
F 1 216 522 0520

IMI TALENT MANAGEMENT
9700 Rockside Road, Suite 410
Cleveland, OH 44125 USA
Contact: Dominick Palazzo / Dennis Boyles
SAG/AFTRA Francised
T 1 216 901 9710
F 1 216 901 9714
W www.imitalent.com
*See Ad This Section

MéLANGE
3130 Mayfield Road, Suite E-308
Cleveland Heights, OH 44118 USA
Contact: Lisa Johnson
T 1 216 371 9710
F 1 216 371 2290

MILLENNIUM MODEL MANAGEMENT
1148 Main Avenue
Cleveland, OH 44113 USA
T 1 216 771 7300
F 1 216 771 8282
W www.millennium-models.com
E tgroman@millennium-models.com
*See Ad Under Virginia Section.

STONE MODEL & TALENT AGENCY
750 W Resource Drive, Suite 200
Cleveland, OH 44131-1836 USA
Contact: Harold Hafner or Miguel DeJesus
T 1 216 351 7300
F 1 216 351 7202
E stonemodels@eastontel.com

Taxi Model Management
1300 W 78th Street
Cleveland, OH 44102 USA
T 1 216 281 8294
F 1 216 281 7243

Tommy's New Attitude
20500 Miles Parkway, Suite 10
Cleveland, OH 44128 USA
T 1 216 475 3388
F 1 216 475 3393

Columbus

CAM TALENT
1350 W 5th Avenue, Suite 25
Columbus, OH 43212 USA
Contact: Carol Mosic
T 1 614 488 1122
F 1 614 488 3895
W www.camtalent.com
E camtalent@aol.com

Jo Goenner Talent Agency
4700 Reed Road, Suite E
Columbus, OH 43220 USA
T 1 614 459 3582
F 1 614 459 3584

John Casablancas/MTM
256 Easton Town Center, Suite C212
Columbus, OH 43219 USA
T 1 614 847 0010
F 1 614 472 2205

John Robert Powers
6412 Sharonwood Boulevard
Columbus, OH 43229 USA
T 1 614 890 0929

The Right Direction Inc
4770 Indianaola Avenue, Suite 160
Columbus, OH 43214 USA
T 1 614 848 3357
F 1 614 848 8748

S2 MANAGEMENT GROUP
844 N High Street
Columbus, OH 43215 USA
Contact: Stephanie Stein
T 1 614 294 0100
F 1 614 294 8281
E S2mgmtgrp@aol.com

Z MODELS
985 Mediterranean Avenue
Columbus, OH 43229 USA
T 1 614 436 9006
F 1 614 436 9016

• • • • • • • • • •

Do It Right
1745 Windsor Street
Cuyahoga Falls, OH 44221 USA
T 1 330 920 0988
F 1 330 920 3791

JO GOENNER TALENT
2299 Miamisburg Centerville Road
Dayton OH 45459 USA
Contact: Jo Goenner
T 1 937 312 0071
F 1 937 312 0081
W www.jogoennertalent.com
E jogoennertalent@erinet.com

SHARKEY AGENCY INC
1299-H Lyons Road
Dayton, OH 45458 USA
Contact: Norma Sharkey, President
T 1 937 434 4461
F 1 937 435 0991

Go International Model Management Inc
3351 Valley View Road NE
Lancaster, OH 43130 USA
T 1 614 554 6974
F 1 740 653 1792

Sherry Lee Finishing School
7745 Cricket Circle NW
Massillion, OH 44646 USA
T 1 330 833 2973

>>

OHIO

John Casablancas/MTM
5405 Southwyck Boulevard, Suite 200
Toledo, OH 43614 USA
T 1 419 866 6335
F 1 419 866 1049

Margaret O'Brien Modeling School
330 S Reynolds Road, Suite 12
Toledo, OH 43615 USA
T 1 419 536 5522
F 1 419 536 5950

Traque International Model Management
901 Washington
Toledo, OH 43624 USA
T 1 419 324 0333
F 1 248 542 6887

MODEL & TALENT AGENCIES

OKLAHOMA

John Casablancas/MTM
107 B.J. Tunnel Boulevard
Miami, OK 74354 USA
T 1 501 444 7972
F 1 501 587 8555

Park Ave Modeling Agency
515 N Canadian Terrace
Mustang, OK 73064-6131 USA
T 1 405 745 9600
F 1 405 745 9505

John Casablancas/MTM
5009 N Pennsylvannia Avenue, Suite 200
Oklahoma City, OK 73112 USA
T 1 405 842 0000
F 1 405 842 0069

HARRISON/GERS MODEL & TALENT AGENCY
1707 W Wilshire Boulevard
Oklahoma City, OK 73116 USA
Contact: Pattye O. Gers
T 1 405 840 4515
T 1 405 840 1546
F 1 405 840 1545

Tulsa

Kirby Casting & Studios
8136A S Harvard Avenue
Tulsa, OK 74137 USA
T 1 918 491 3410
F 1 918 494 6844

LINDA LAYMAN AGENCY LTD
3546 East 51st Street
Tulsa, OK 74135-3518 USA
Contact: Linda Layman & Don Hull
T 1 918 744 0888
F 1 918 744 1802
E laymanagcy@juno.com

RUSSELL LANGLEY AGENCY
309 E 2nd Street
Tulsa, OK 74120 USA
Contact: Lisa Staton, Director
T 1 918 749 5533
F 1 918 749 5549
W www.langleyagency.com
E langleyagency@yahoo.com

SCOUT TEAM
A DIVISION OF AGENCY, TALENT & MODELS
8137 E 63rd Place, Suite C
Tulsa, OK 74133 USA
Contact: Andrew York, President
T 1 918 250 5909
F 1 918 250 5492

MODEL & TALENT AGENCIES

OREGON

John Casablancas/MTM
9400 SW Beaverton Hillsdale Highway, Suite 130
Beaverton, OR 97005 USA
T 1 503 297 7730
F 1 503 292 8772

ABC Kids & Teens
1144 Willagillespie Road, Suite 1
Eugene, OR 97401 USA
T 1 541 485 6960
F 1 541 485 1994

Unlimited Models & Talent Agency
P.O. Box 12086
Eugene, OR 97401 USA
T 1 541 683 9323
F 1 541 684 9125

IMD • IMAGE & MODELING DEVELOPMENT
1245 N Riverside Drive, Suite 20
Medford, OR 97501 USA
Contact: Teresa Farmen
T 1 541 858 8158
F 1 541 858 1975
W www.imdmodeling.com
E info@imdmodeling.com

SOUL MANAGEMENT
735 Alder Street
Medford, OR 97501 USA
Contact: Tia
T 1 541 858 2777

Portland

ABC MODEL/TALENT/SPORT MANAGEMENT
3829 NE Tillamook
Portland, OR 97212 USA
Contact: Carol Lukens
T 1 503 249 2945
F 1 503 249 7429
E abcknt@teleport.com

CUSICKS' TALENT AGENCY
1009 N.W. Hoyt, Suite 100
Portland, OR 97209 USA
Contact: Justin Habel
Fashion print and runway, commercial print & on-camera
T 1 503 274 8555
F 1 503 274 4615
W www.q6talent.com
E justin@q6talent.com

FACE VALUE MODEL & TALENT
418 SW Washington Street, Suite 400
Portland, OR 97204 USA
Contact: Ronnie
T 1 503 517 8691
F 1 503 517 8780
***See Ad This Section.**

Mode Models
319 SW Washington, Suite 719
Portland, OR 97204 USA
T 1 503 227 6633
F 1 503 243 5327

RYAN ARTISTS INC
239 NW 13th Avenue, Suite 215
Portland, OR 97209 USA
Contact: Kit Just
T 1 503 274 1005
F 1 503 274 0907
W www.ryanartists.com
E kit@ryanartists.com

CINDERELLA MODELS AGENCY
317 Court NE, Suite 200
Salem, OR 97301 USA
Contact: Sue Ferguson, Owner
T 1 503 581 1073
F 1 503 581 2260
W www.cinderellamodels.com

MODEL & TALENT AGENCIES

PENNSYLVANIA

PRO MODEL & TALENT MANAGEMENT
1244 Hamilton Street, 2nd Floor
Allentown, PA 18102 USA
Contact: Laurie Bickford
T 1 610 820 5359
F 1 610 434 0900
W www.promodelagency.com
E promodel@fast.net

Barbizon
22 Greenfield Avenue
Ardmore, PA 19003 USA
T 1 610 649 9700
F 1 610 645 9621

Slickis Models
1777 Walton Road, Suite 204
Blue Bell, PA 19422 USA
T 1 215 540 0440
F 1 215 957 6285

Kane Modeling School & Agency
110 Morgan Center
Butler, PA 16001 USA
T 1 724 287 0576

Look Model Management
Highway 315, 228 Main Street
Dupont, PA 18641 USA
T 1 570 655 7220
F 1 570 655 7221

>>

Vision Model Management
5120 West Ridge Road
Erie, PA 16506 USA
T 1 814 833 7346
F 1 814 922 7740

Barbizon
1033 Maclay Street, P.O. Box 5445
Harrisburg, PA 17110 USA
T 1 717 234 3277
F 1 717 234 4369

FASHION MYSTIQUE MODELING AGENCY
611 N Mountain Road
Harrisburg, PA 17112 USA
Contact: Dawn Lackner
T 1 717 561 2099
F 1 717 909 9987
W www.fashionmystiquemodeling.com
E fashmys@earthlink.net

MILLENNIUM MODEL MANAGEMENT
601 S Henderson Road, Suite 203
King of Prussia, PA 19406 USA
Contact: Linda Vetter
T 1 610 337 8450
F 1 610 337 8470

Plaza 7 Model & Talent Reps
160 North Gulph Road
King of Prussia, PA 19406 USA
T 1 610 337 2693
F 1 610 337 4762

BOWMAN AGENCY
P.O. Box 4071
Lancaster, PA 17604 USA
Contact: Mary Bowman, Owner
T 1 717 898 7716
F 1 717 898 6084
E mlbowman@thebowmanagency.com

John Casablancas/MTM
P.O. Box 670
Langhorne, PA 19047 USA
T 1 215 752 8600
F 1 215 752 8946

MMA • MODEL MANAGEMENT AGENCY INC
106 S Bellevue Avenue, Suite 212
Langhorne, PA 19047 USA
Contact: Ellen Wasser-Hrin
FULL SERVICE AGENCY SERVING TRI-STATE AREA
Places models internationally; Also available for national bookings.
T 1 215 752 8603
F 1 215 752 8604

MILLENIA MODEL & TALENT MANAGEMENT
4902 Carlisle Pike, Suite 228
Mechanicsburg, PA 17055 USA
Contact: Kelli Harman
T 1 717 730 4075
F 1 717 730 4073
E rtklharman@aol.com

MAIN LINE MODELS
1215 West Baltimore Pike, Suite 9
Media, PA 19063 USA
Contact: Laraine Colden
T 1 610 565 5445
F 1 610 891 9140
E mlmtalent@compuserve.com

John Robert Powers
1528 Spruce Street
Philadelphia, PA 19102 USA
T 1 215 732 4060
F 1 215 732 6212

ON TRACK MODELING INC
4190 City Avenue, Suite 528
Philadelphia, PA 19131 USA
T 1 215 877 4500
F 1 215 877 6457
***See Ad This Section.**

REINHARD MODEL & TALENT AGENCY
2021 Arch Street, Suite 400
Philadelphia, PA 19103 USA
Contact: Virginia B. Doyle
T 1 215 567 2000
F 1 215 567 6322
W www.reinhardagency.com

Pittsburgh

Barbizon
9 Parkway Center, Suite 160
Pittsburgh, PA 15220 USA
T 1 412 937 0700
F 1 412 937 0704

DOCHERTY MODEL & TALENT
109 Market Street
Pittsburgh, PA 15222 USA
Contact: Debra L. Docherty, President
PRINT • FILM • TELEVISION • RADIO
RUNWAY • PROMOTIONAL
T 1 412 765 1400
F 1 412 765 0403
E docherty@sgi.net

MTM / Model & Talent Management
394 Rodi Road
Pittsburgh, PA 15235 USA
T 1 412 731 7171
F 1 412 731 5636

Prestige Modeling Agency
10028 Frankstown Road
Pittsburgh, PA 15235 USA
T 1 412 731 4810
F 1 412 731 8970

THE TALENT GROUP INC
2820 Smallman Street
Pittsburgh, PA 15222 USA
Contact: Richard Kohn
Print • TV • Film • Promotional
Runway • Trade Shows
T 1 412 471 8011
F 1 412 471 0875
E talent@usaor.net
***See Ad This Section.**

>>

PENNSYLVANIA

VAN ENTERPRISES AGENCY
908 Perry Highway, Suite 1
Pittsburgh, PA 15229 USA
Contact: Laurie Ann Vangenewitt
Representing Children, Teens, Adults & Senior Citizens
T 1 412 364 0411
F 1 412 931 4424

• • • • • • • • • •

DONATELLI MODELING & CASTING AGENCY
156 Madison Avenue, Hyde Park
Reading, PA 19605-2962 USA
Contact: Tony or Mickey Donatelli
T 1 610 921 0777
F 1 610 921 0778
W www.donatellimodels.com
E tony@donatellimodels.com

Mary Leister Charm & Finishing School
539 Court Street
Reading, PA 19601 USA
T 1 610 373 6150

Click Models
216 Green Tree Street
West Chester, PA 19382 USA
T 1 610 399 0700
F 1 610 399 3004

MODEL & TALENT AGENCIES

PUERTO RICO

D'ROSE INTERNATIONAL
1261 Ponce de Leon Avenue
San Juan, PR 00907 USA
Contact: Ms. Rose Perez, President
T 1 787 722 5580
F 1 787 724 1735
W www.droseintl.com
E drose@coqui.net

Unica
Calle Cesar Gonzalez No. 400, Depto. 157
San Juan, 00918 USA
T 1 787 756 7834
F 1 787 250 6463

Visage International Models
P.O. Box 30675
San Juan, 00929-1675 USA
T 1 787 292 2582
F 1 787 292 2582

MODEL & TALENT AGENCIES

RHODE ISALND

A.K.A. Models
239 Harris Avenue, 2nd Floor
Providence, RI 02903 USA
T 1 401 751 8300
F 1 401 831 9160

MODEL CLUB INC
355 S Water Street
Providence, RI 02903 USA
Contact: Ed Sliney
Call for Agency Book...
Will Overnight Express Immediately.
T 1 401 273 7120
F 1 401 273 1642
W www.modelclubinc.com
E modelclubinc@worldnet.att.net

Rhode Island Casting Services
P.O. Box A
Rumford, RI 02916 USA
T 1 401 941 5500
F 1 508 336 0826

Character Kids Model Management
1645 Warwick Avenue, Suite 225
Warwick, RI 02889 USA
T 1 401 739 3334
F 1 401 732 8188

John Casablancas/MTM
1 Lambert Lind Highway
Warwick, RI 02888 USA
T 1 401 463 5866
F 1 401 463 8504

NINE MANAGEMENT
1645 Warwick Avenue, Suite 225
Warwick, RI 02889 USA
T 1 401 732 8487
F 1 401 732 8406
W www.ninemanagement.com
E ninemgt1@msn.com

MODEL & TALENT AGENCIES

SOUTH CAROLINA

CD MODELS & PROMOTIONS
1396 Stiles Bee Avenue
Charleston, SC 29412 USA
Contact: Cory Dueger, President
T 1 843 762 6655
E duegercory@hotmail.com

MILLIE LEWIS MODELS & TALENT
1904 Savannah Highway
Charleston, SC 29407 USA
Contact: Suzanne Manseau Green, Owner/Director
T 1 843 571 7781
F 1 843 763 0365
W www.mlamtc.com
E mlcharleston@hotmail.com

CAROLINA WINDS PRODUCTIONS
141 Gadsden Street
Chester, SC 29706 USA
Contact: Donna Ehrlich
T 1 803 581 2278
F 1 803 581 7703

COLLINS MODELS & TALENT INC
1410 Colonial Life Building, Suite 230
Columbia, SC 29210 USA
Contact: Diane Turok / Larry Baldwin
Mailing: P.O. Box 234, Columbia, SC 29202
T 1 803 216 0550
T 1 803 345 1364
F 1 803 932 9285
W www.collinsmodels.com
E collinsmodels@aol.com

MILLIE LEWIS MODEL & TALENT AGENCY
3612 Landmark Drive, Suite D
Columbia, SC 29204 USA
Contact: Sheilah Dixon, Director
T 1 803 782 7338
F 1 803 790 0444

Shaw's Model & Talent Center
200 Berkshire Drive
Columbia, SC 29223 USA
T 1 803 699 0158

DREAMS UNLIMITED
959 Mauldin Road, Suite 104
Greenville, SC 29607 USA
Contact: Pam Peters
T 1 864 299 5077
T 1 864 299 5075 Recording Studio
F 1 864 299 5079
E scagent4u@aol.com

MILLIE LEWIS MODEL/TALENT AGENCY • GREENVILLE
1228 S Pleasantburg Drive
Greenville, SC 29605 USA
Contact: Barbara & George Corell
T 1 864 299 1101
F 1 864 299 1119
E gcorell@acsinc.net

Carolina Modeling Agency
722 Antler Ridge Cove
Myrtle Beach, SC 29579 USA
T 1 843 236 3822
F 1 843 236 3439

ASA International Model & Talent Management
3926 Wesley Street, Studio 702
Myrtle Beach, SC 29579 USA
T 1 843 236 8445

Betty Lane Models & Talent
951 Doyle Street
Orangeburg, SC 29115 USA
T 1 803 534 9672
F 1 803 535 3000

SHOWCASE MODELS & TALENT
1200 33rd Avenue S
North Myrtle Beach, SC 29582 USA
Contact: Marsha McCollum, Owner
T 1 843 272 8009
F 1 843 361 0253
W www.showcasetalent.com
E marsha@showcasetalent.com

RUSSELL ADAIR FASHION STUDIO
1418 D Avenue
West Columbia, SC 29169 USA
Photography, Stylist, M/U, Wardrobe
Contact: Russell Adair
T 1 803 794 7233

MODEL & TALENT AGENCIES

SOUTH DAKOTA

Haute Models
1002 W 6th Street
Sioux Falls, SD 57104 USA
T 1 605 334 6110

Professional Image By Rosemary
2815 East 26th Street
Sioux Falls, SD 57103 USA
T 1 605 334 0619
F 1 605 334 1407

MODEL & TALENT AGENCIES

TENNESSEE

The Hurd Agency
500 Eversholt Court
Antioch, TN 37013 USA
T 1 615 399 9901
F 1 615 365 0246 Gregory James

ADVANTAGE MODEL & TALENT
P.O. Box 3145
Brentwood, TN 37024 USA
Contact: Nise Davies
SAG & AFTRA Franchised
T 1 615 833 3005
F 1 615 331 8267
E advantage@datatek.com

Finesse Modeling Agency & Talent Mgmt
112 Briscoe Circle
Bristol, TN 37620 USA
T 1 888 870 7504

Ambiance Models & Talent
1096 Dayton Boulevard
Chattanooga, TN 37415 USA
T 1 423 265 2121
F 1 423 265 2190

Career Model & Talent Management
P.O. Box 977
Hendersonville, TN 37077 USA
T 1 615 824 1622
F 1 615 824 1611

Brenda Wilson Modeling School & Management
2600 Fort Henry Drive
Kingsport, TN 37664 USA
T 1 423 246 6838
F 1 423 246 6838

Knoxville

18 KARAT TALENT & MODELING AGENCY
6409 Deane Hill Drive,
Knoxville, TN 37919-6003 USA
Contact: Cindy Swicegood
T 1 865 558 0004
F 1 865 558 9823
W www.18karat.com
E cindy@18karat.com

Knoxville Model Agency
433 Kendall Road
Knoxville, TN 37919 USA
T 1 865 693 6010
F 1 865 588 6922

Premier Model & Talent Agency
5201 Kingston Pike, Suite 6-320
Knoxville, TN 37919 USA
T 1 865 588 8083
F 1 865 588 1806

TALENT TREK AGENCY
406 11th Street
Knoxville, TN 37916 USA
Contact: Charlotte Dennison / Juanell Walker
T 1 865 977 8735
F 1 865 977 9200
W www.talentrek.com
E talentrek@aol.com

Memphis

COLORS AGENCY INC
408 South Front Street, Suite 108
Memphis, TN 38103 USA
Contact: Annette A. Outlan / Jo W. Bracey
T 1 901 523 9900
F 1 901 523 2050
W www.colorsagency.com
E info@colorsagency.com

THE DONNA GROFF AGENCY INC
P.O. Box 382517
Memphis, TN 38183-2517 USA
Contact: Donna Groff
T 1 901 854 5561
F 1 901 854 5561

John Casablancas/MTM
5028 Park Avenue
Memphis, TN 38117 USA
T 1 901 685 0066
F 1 901 685 0077

OUR AGENCY
1441 Jackson Avenue
Memphis, TN 38107 USA
Contact: Autumn Chastain, Director
or Chad Johnson, Model Division
T 1 901 278 0328
F 1 901 278 0328
W www.ouragencyofmemphis.com
E info@ouragencyofmemphis.com

Robbins Model & Talent
176 Walnut Bend
Memphis, TN 38018 USA
T 1 901 753 8360
F 1 901 754 0902

Nashville

AMAX-Amer'n Models, Actors, Extras
4121 Hillsboro Road, Hillsboro Corner, Suite 300
Nashville, TN 37215 USA
T 1 615 292 0246
F 1 615 292 2054

Billy Deaton Talent
1300 Divison Street, Suite 102
Nashville, TN 37203 USA
T 1 615 244 4259
F 1 615 242 1177

Capitol Management & Talent Group
1300 Division Street
Nashville, TN 37203 USA
T 1 615 244 2440
F 1 615 242 1177

COLEMAN MODEL & TALENT AGENCY
P.O. Box 40191
Nashville, TN 37204 USA
Contact: Crystal Coleman / Cindy Lovell
T 1 615 385 5797
F 1 615 269 3386

HARPER/SPEER AGENCY INC
P.O. Box 158779
Nashville, TN 37215 USA
Contact: Suzan K. Speer
T 1 615 383 1455
F 1 615 383 5464
E harpspeer@aol.com
***See Ad This Section.**

IMAGE PLUS INTERNATIONAL
1300 Division Street, Suite 200
Nashville, TN 37203 USA
Contact: Kimberly Ann Cook
T 1 931 224 1059
F 1 615 242 1177
E Kimberly@imageplusinternational.com

Jo-Susan Modeling & Finishing School
2817 W End Avenue, Suite 210
Nashville, TN 37203 USA
T 1 615 327 8726
F 1 615 356 9483

Lynda Alexander & Associates
315 Arbor Creek Boulevard
Nashville, TN 37217 USA
T 1 615 367 9398
F 1 615 367 9398

TALENT TREK • NASHVILLE
2021 21st Avenue S, Suite 102
Nashville, TN 37212 USA
Contact: Evelyn Foster / Sharon Smith
T 1 615 279 0010
F 1 615 279 0013
W www.talentrek.com
E ttanash@aol.com

TML Talent Agency
P.O. Box 40763
Nashville, TN 37204 USA
T 1 615 321 5596
F 1 615 321 5497

≫

William Morris Agency
2100 W End Avenue, Suite 1000
Nashville, TN 37203 USA
T 1 615 963 3000
F 1 615 963 3090

MODEL & TALENT AGENCIES

TEXAS

Tomas Agency
14275 Midway Road, Suite 220
Addison, TX 75001 USA
T 1 972 687 9181
F 1 972 687 9182

Anderson Model & Talent
2722 W 6th Street
Amarillo, TX 79106 USA
T 1 806 374 1159
F 1 806 374 2420

DIANE DICK INTERNATIONAL MODELING & TALENT AGENCY
1410 S Washington Street
Amarillo, TX 79102 USA
Contact: Diane Dick
T 1 806 376 8736
F 1 806 376 8841
E Ddleg@aol.com

MODELS WEST MODEL & TALENT AGENCY
3405 South Western, Suite 201
Amarillo, TX 79109 USA
Contact: Carol Henderson
T 1 806 352 1943
F 1 806 355 6154
W www.ModelsWest.com
E modelswest@aol.com

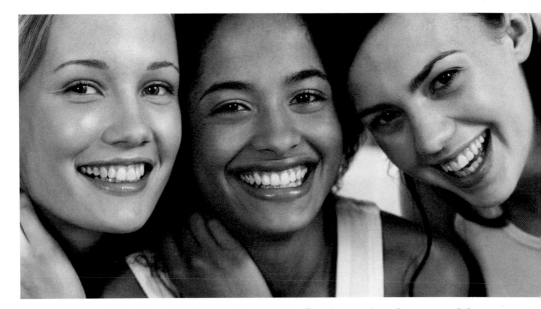

Austin

ACCLAIM TALENT
4107 Medical Parkway, Suite 210
Austin, TX 78756 USA
Contact: Jeff Nightbyrd / Steve Birmingham
T 1 512 323 5566
F 1 512 323 5553
W www.acclaimtalent.com
E acclaim@jump.net

DB Talent
3107 Slaughter Lane W
Austin, TX 78748-5705 USA
T 1 512 292 1030
F 1 512 292 1032

John Robert Powers
9037 Research Boulevard, Suite 100
Austin, TX 78759 USA
T 1 512 835 5089

K Hall Agency
700 Rio Grande
Austin, TX 78701 USA
T 1 512 476 7523
F 1 512 476 7544

• • • • • • • • • •

REFLECTIONS FASHION & TALENT AGENCY INC
110 Alta Plaza
Corpus Christi, TX 78411 USA
Contact: Doreen Crow, Owner/Director
T 1 361 854 9277
F 1 361 857 5447
E dcrow@caller.infi.net

Dallas

Barbizon School
12700 Hillcrest Road, Suite 142
Dallas, TX 75230-2009 USA
T 1 972 980 7477
F 1 972 934 0941

THE CAMPBELL AGENCY
3906 Lemmon Avenue, Suite 200
Dallas, TX 75219 USA
Contact: Nancy Campbell
T 1 214 522 8991
F 1 214 522 8997

CLIPSE MANAGEMENT INC
1420 W Mockingbird Lane, Suite 280
Dallas, TX 75247 USA
T 1 214 634 4950
F 1 214 634 4955
W www.clipsemanagement.com

DALLAS MODEL GROUP
12700 Hillcrest Road, Suite 142
Dallas, TX 75230 USA
Contact: SM Stephan
T 1 972 980 7647
F 1 972 934 0941
E dmgmaai@hotmail.com

GANSON MODEL MANAGEMENT
6434 Maple Avenue, Suite 336
Dallas, TX 75235 USA
Contact: Eric L. Ganison
T 1 214 366 2412
F 1 214 366 0376
W www.gansonmodelmanagement.com
E milan@airmail.net

>>

KIM DAWSON AGENCY INC
2300 Stemmons Freeway, 1643 Apparel Mart
Dallas, TX 75258 USA
Mailing Address: PO Box 585060, Dallas, TX 75258 USA
TX Lic#: TA 115
T 1 214 638 2414
F 1 214 638 7567
***See Ad This Section.**

KIM DAWSON AGENCY INC • TALENT DIVISION
2710 N Stemmons Freeway, Suite 700
Dallas, TX 75207 USA
TX Lic#: TA 216
T 1 214 630 5161
F 1 214 630 8259
***See Ad This Section.**

THE KIMBERLY ELLIS GROUP
8204 Elmbrook, Suite 201
Dallas, TX 75247 USA
Contact: Kimberly Ellis, Chairman/CEO
T 1 214 638 2020
F 1 214 638 2048
W www.thekimberlyellisgroup.com

ON TRACK MODELING INC
Contact: Michael Mercer
T 1 817 838 3770
***See Ad This Section.**

PAGE PARKES MODELS REP • PAGE 214
3303 Lee Parkway, Suite 205
Dallas, TX 75219 USA
Contact: Nancy Halford
TX Lic#: TA 242
T 1 214 526 4434
F 1 214 526 6034
W www.page305.com
E dallasmodels@pageparkes.com

Marquee Talent Inc
5911 Maple Avenue, P.O. Box 35269
Dallas, TX 75235 USA
T 1 214 357 0355
F 1 214 357 0442

Mary Collins Agency
2909 Cole Avenue, Suite 250
Dallas, TX 75204 USA
T 1 214 871 8900
F 1 214 871 8945

Peggy Taylor Talent Inc
1825 Market Center Boulevard, Suite 320
Dallas, TX 75207 USA
T 1 214 651 7884
F 1 214 651 7329

Rody Kent & Associates
P.O. Box 140857
Dallas, TX 75214 USA
T 1 214 827 3418
F 1 214 827 2429

THE WILLIAM WARE AGENCY
2931 Irving Blvd, Suite 100
Dallas, TX 75247 USA
Contact: Bill Ware
T 1 214 638 6200
F 1 214 638 6273
W www.williamwareagency.com
E bill@williamwareagency.com

• • • • • • • • • •

The Talent House
812 North Virginia, Suite 200
El Paso, TX 79902 USA
T 1 915 533 1945
F 1 915 533 1953

John Robert Powers
6320 Camp Bowie Boulevard
Ft Worth, TX 76116 USA
T 1 817 738 2021
F 1 817 738 2029

Premier Talent
P.O. Box 532788
Grand Prairie, TX 75053 USA
T 1 972 237 1919
F 1 972 237 1616

Houston

ACTORS ETC INC
2620 Fountain View, Suite 210
Houston, TX 77057 USA
Contact: Denise Coburn, President
T 1 713 785 4495
F 1 713 785 2641
W www.actoretc.com
E actoretc@insync.net

BARBIZON • HOUSTON
5433 Westheimer Road, Suite 300
Houston, TX 77056 USA
Contact: Gail Barry, President
TX Lic#: TA 00000153
T 1 713 850 9111
F 1 713 850 8229
W www.barbizonhouston.com
E barbizon@barbizonhouston.com

>>

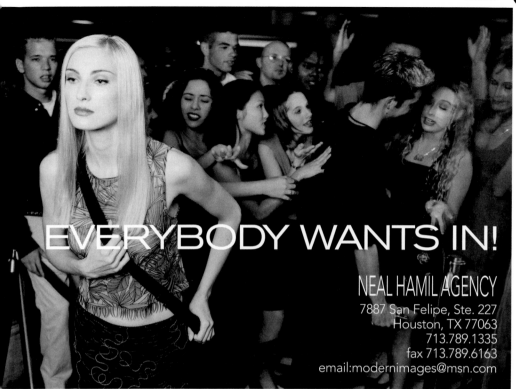

Chris Wilson's Studio for Actors
2506 South Boulevard
Houston, TX 77098 USA
T 1 713 520 1991
F 1 713 520 1993

FIRST MODELS & TALENT AGENCY
5433 Westheimer Avenue, Suite 310
Houston, TX 77056 USA
Contact: Gail Barry, President
TX Lic#: TA 00000153
T 1 713 850 9611
F 1 713 850 8229
E firstmodels@firstmodelshouston.com

INTERMEDIA / PAGE 713 MODEL & TALENT AGENCY
2727 Kirby Drive, Penthouse
Houston, TX 77098 USA
Contact: Page Parkes-Eveleth
TX Lic#: TA 117
T 1 713 807 8222
F 1 713 807 0055
W www.pageparkes.com
E houstonmodels@pageparkes.com

MAYO HILL SCHOOL OF MODELING
7887 San Felipe, Suite 227
Houston, TX 77063 USA
TX Lic#: TA 00000304
T 1 713 789 7340
F 1 713 789 6163
W www.mayohill.com
E modernimages@msn.com
***See Ad This Section.**

NEAL HAMIL AGENCY
7887 San Felipe, Suite 227
Houston, TX 77063 USA
Contact: BJ Shell or Jeff Shell
Print & Fashion Bookings, Broadcast Talents
TX Lic#: TA 00000304
T 1 713 789 1335
F 1 713 789 6163
E modernimages@msn.com
***See Ad This Section.**

PAGE PARKES CENTER OF MODELING & ACTING
2727 Kirby Drive, 8th Floor
Houston, TX 77098 USA
Contact: Lisa Lyngos
T 1 713 807 8200
F 1 713 807 0022
W www.pageparkes.com
E modelcenter@pageparkes.com

Pastorini-Bosby Talent Agency
3013 Fountainview Drive
Houston, TX 77057-6120 USA
T 1 713 266 4488
F 1 713 266 3314

SHERRY YOUNG/MAD HATTER MODEL & TALENT AGENCY
2620 Fountainview, Suite 212
Houston, TX 77057 USA
Contact: Michael Young, Owner
T 1 713 266 5800
F 1 713 266 2044
E symhtalent@aol.com

• • • • • • • • • •

PS Images
1105 Pueblo Drive
Midland, TX 79705 USA
T 1 915 683 0844
F 1 915 683 0870

Teresa Models & Company
701 E Plano Parkway, Suite 409
Plano, TX 75074-6757 USA
T 1 972 943 3471
F 1 972 943 3472

San Antonio

Avant Models & Casting Inc
85 NE Loop 410, Suite 218A
San Antonio, TX 78216 USA
T 1 210 308 8411
F 1 210 308 8412

CALLIOPE TALENT, MODEL & ARTIST MANAGEMENT LLC
1802 NE Loop 410, Suite 107
San Antonio, TX 78217 USA
Contact: Kristy Martin, Owner/Director
TX Lic#: TA 275
T 1 210 804 1055
F 1 210 804 2008
W www.calliopetalent.com
E CalliopeSA@aol.com

Condra/Artista Model & Talent Agency
13300 Old Blanco Road
San Antonio, TX 78216 USA
T 1 210 492 9947
F 1 210 492 9921

Jeska Model Management
115 Tabard
San Antonio, TX 78213-3918 USA
T 1 800 451 5813
F 1 800 236 7071

Linda Woods Modeling Agency
14100 San Pedro Avenue, Suite 611
San Antonio, TX 78232 USA
T 1 210 340 5423
F 1 210 490 4914

• • • • • • • • • •

John Robert Powers
1828 ESE Loop 323, Suite R1B
Tyler, TX 75701 USA
T 1 903 531 2240
F 1 903 531 2250

MODEL & TALENT AGENCIES

US VIRGIN ISLANDS

Cyndee's Models in the Isle
P.O. Box 8600, Sunny Isle
St Croix, 00823 USA
T 1 340 713 9148

C9 INTERNATIONAL MODELS
P.O. Box 573
St Croix, VI 00821 US Virgin Islands
Contact: Ben Mitchell
T 1 340 778 1015
F 1 340 778 1015
W www.c9internationalmodels.com
E ben_123@hotmail.com

MODEL & TALENT AGENCIES

UTAH

Salt Lake City

Executive Model Shop
2900 S State Street, Suite 300
Salt Lake City, UT 84115 USA
T 1 801 487 2799
F 1 801 487 2806

John Robert Powers
2733 E Parley's Way, Suite 204
Salt Lake City, UT 84109 USA
T 1 801 412 0900
F 1 801 412 0565

MCCARTY AGENCY INC
1326 Foothill Boulevard
Salt Lake City, UT 84108-2321 USA
Contact: Susie McCarty
T 1 801 581 9292
F 1 801 581 0921
W www.mccartyagency.com
E smccarty@uswest.net

>>

METCALF MODELING & TALENT AGENCY
Contact: Bonnie Metcalf
T 1 800 820 8777
E metcalfagt@aol.com
International Placement & Development

PULSE MANAGEMENT
175 W 2700 South
Salt Lake City, UT 84101 USA
Contact: Vikki Leza
Mailing: P.O. Box 651208, SLC, UT 84165-1208
T 1 801 328 4546
T 1 888 727 6559
F 1 801 328 4546
W www.pulsemanagement.com
E vikki@juno.com

TALENT MANAGEMENT GROUP INC
339 E 3900 South
Salt Lake City, UT 84107 USA
Contact: Vickie Panek • Linda Bearman
T 1 801 263 6940
F 1 801 263 6950
W www.talentmg.com

URBAN MODEL & FILM MANAGEMENT INC
566 North 300 West
Salt Lake City, UT 84103 USA
Contact: Tina Bullen
Print, Runway, Live Promotion, Commercial/Film
T 1 801 539 0800
F 1 801 539 0844
W www.urbantalent.com
E tbullen@urbantalent.com
*See Ad This Section.

MODEL & TALENT AGENCIES

VERMONT

Debra Lewin Productions & Talent
269 Pearl Street, Suite 2
Burlington, VT 05401 USA
T 1 802 865 2234
F 1 802 865 8327

MODEL & TALENT AGENCIES

VIRGINIA

ENCORE! MODEL AND TALENT AGENCY INC
17 Keith's Lane
Alexandria, VA 22314 USA
Contact: Jeannie Kincer Reinke
Trade Shows/Promotions, Nationwide!
T 1 703 548 0900
F 1 703 549 8278

Model & Talent Management
249 S Van Dorn, Suite 210
Alexandria, VA 22304 USA
T 1 703 823 5200
F 1 703 751 2531

PARRIS INC
218 N Lee Street, Suite 200
Alexandria, VA 22314 USA
Contact: Chandra Parris
Event Planning, Coordination & Promotion Services
T 1 703 837 8889
F 1 703 837 9599
*See Ad This Section.

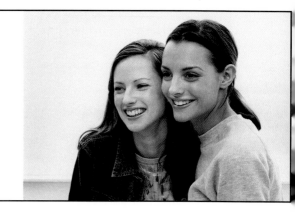

MODEL X AGENCY
P.O. Box 6794
Arlington, VA 22206 USA
Contact: Jennifer Bossard
T 1 703 314 4761
E mxagency@hotmail.com

ON CALL MODELS & TALENT
946 Ferryman Quay
Chesapeake, VA 23323 USA
Contact: Carol Jo & Ron Gustafson
T 1 757 485 1201
F 1 757 558 0556
W www.oncallmodels.com

Jackie Fenderson
1224 West Roslyn Road
Colonial Heights, VA 23834 USA
T 1 804 526 7347

MODEL SOURCE INC
601 Caroline Street, Suite 204
Fredericksburg, VA 22401 USA
Contact: Heather Cole, Director
T 1 540 374 1935
F 1 540 374 1941
E modlsource@aol.com

JUDY GIBSON AND ASSOCIATES
J.G. MODEL MANAGEMENT
40 Channel Lane
Hampton, VA 23664 USA
Contact: Judy Gibson, Director/Photographer
T 1 757 850 8808
F 1 757 850 4121
E judygibson@rcn.com

Ann L School of Modeling
1925 East Market Street, Suite 354
Harrisonburg, VA 22801 USA
T 1 540 434 6664
F 1 540 289 5762

BONNIE ADLEMAN AGENCY
2600 Robious Crossing Drive
Midlothian, VA 23113 USA
T 1 804 379 8200
F 1 804 379 8221
E bonatalent@aol.com
E mail@bonnieagency.com

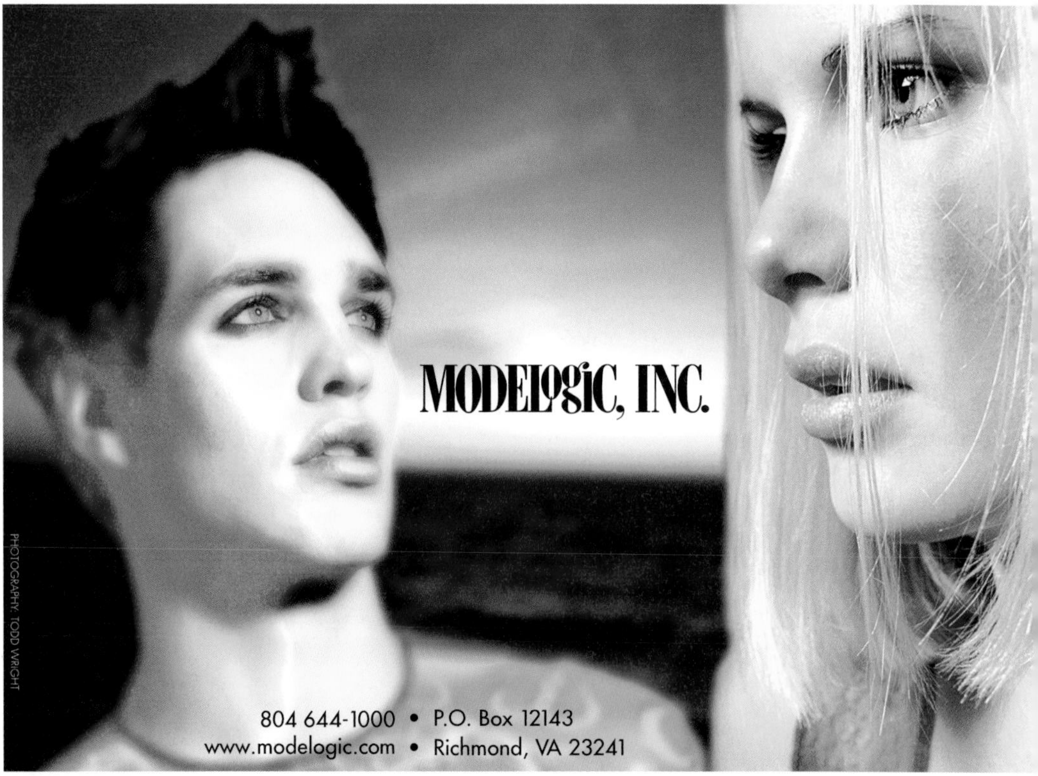

WRIGHT MODEL & TALENT AGENCY
12638-16 Jefferson Avenue
Newport News, VA 23602 USA
Contact: Pat Wright
T 1 757 886 5884
F 1 757 886 9128
E wrightma@hrfn.net

MODELOGIC INC
2501 E Broad Street
Richmond, VA 23223 USA
Contact: Stacie Vanchieri, President
T 1 804 644 1000
F 1 804 644 0051
W www.modelogic.com
E stacie@modelogic.com
***See Ad This Section.**

Winning Image Models
8805 Millwood Drive
Spotsylvania, VA 221553 USA
T 1 540 582 2890
F 1 540 720 4643

MILLENNIUM MODEL MANAGEMENT
8321 Old Courthouse Road, Suite 251
Vienna, VA 22182 USA
Contact: Terry Groman
T 1 703 903 0040
F 1 703 903 0045
W www.millennium-models.com
E tgroman@millennium-models.com
***See Ad This Section.**

New Faces Models
8230 Leesburg Pike, Suite 520
Vienna, VA 22182 USA
T 1 703 821 0786
F 1 703 821 1129

Evie Mansfield Modeling
505 S Independence Boulevard, Suite 205
Virginia Beach, VA 23452 USA
T 1 757 490 5990
F 1 757 499 4742

Steinhart/Norton Agency
312 Arctic Crescent
Virginia Beach, VA 23451-3415 USA
T 1 757 422 8535
F 1 757 422 8752

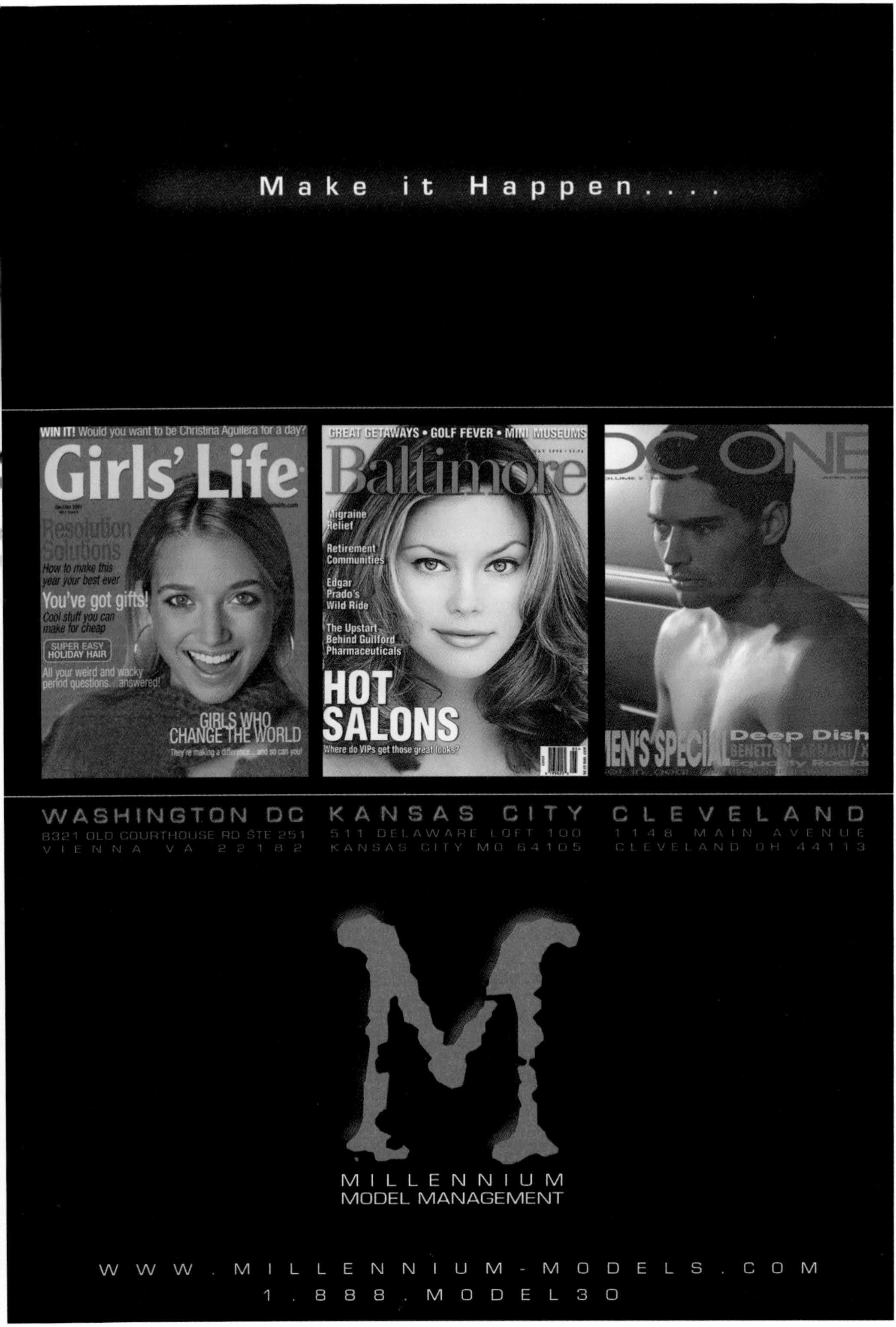
Make it Happen....
WIN IT! Would you want to be Christina Aguilera for a day?
Girls' Life
Resolution Solutions
How to make this year your best ever
You've got gifts!
Cool stuff you can make for cheap
SUPER EASY HOLIDAY HAIR
All your weird and wacky period questions...answered!
GIRLS WHO CHANGE THE WORLD
They're making a difference...and so can you!
GREAT GETAWAYS • GOLF FEVER • MINI MUSEUMS
Baltimore
Migraine Relief
Retirement Communities
Edgar Prado's Wild Ride
The Upstart Behind Guilford Pharmaceuticals
HOT SALONS
Where do VIPs get those great looks?
DC ONE
MEN'S SPECIAL
Deep Dish
BENETTON ARMANI/X
WASHINGTON DC
8321 OLD COURTHOUSE RD STE 251
VIENNA VA 22182
KANSAS CITY
511 DELAWARE LOFT 100
KANSAS CITY MO 64105
CLEVELAND
1148 MAIN AVENUE
CLEVELAND OH 44113
MILLENNIUM
MODEL MANAGEMENT
WWW.MILLENNIUM-MODELS.COM
1.888.MODEL30

MODEL & TALENT AGENCIES

WASHINGTON

John Casablancas/MTM
50 116th Avenue SE, Suite 100
Bellevue, WA 98004 USA
T 1 425 646 3585
F 1 425 637 9461

SHARON'S MODEL & TALENT AGENCY & MANAGEMENT
5458 Chico Way
Bremerton, WA 98312 USA
Contact: Sharon Johnson
T 1 360 308 8876
F 1 360 308 8876
W www.sharonsmodels.com
E touchtime1@netzero.com

NFI Models/Northwest Kids
19009 33rd Avenue W, Suite 100
Lynnwood, WA 98036 USA
T 1 425 775 8385
F 1 425 771 1114

AMI • ANDERSEN MODELS INTERNATIONAL
1302 28th Avenue Court
Milton, WA 98354 USA
Contact: Chuck Andersen, Owner/Director
Seattle-Based, N.A.M.A. affiliated agency focused on scouting & developing models for world-wide promotion.
T 1 253 952 2002
F 1 253 952 8816
E cande98752@aol.com

Alleinad-The Total Image
147 N Rogers
Olympia, WA 98502 USA
T 1 360 705 2573
F 1 360 705 3889

Seattle

ABC MODEL/TALENT/SPORT MANAGEMENT
10415 NE 37th Circle, Bldg 4
Seattle, WA 98033 USA
Contact: David Van Maren
A Full Service Management Company with offices in Los Angeles, Portland, Eugene & Seattle.
T 1 425 822 6339
F 1 425 822 5457

Actors Group
603 Stewart Street, Suite 214
Seattle, WA 98101 USA
T 1 206 624 9465
F 1 206 624 9466

Barbizon
1501 4th Avenue, Suite 305
Seattle, WA 98101 USA
T 1 206 223 1500
F 1 206 624 7091

HEFFNER MANAGEMENT
Westlake Tower, 1601 Fifth Avenue, Suite 2301
Seattle, WA 98101 USA
Contact: Marsha Ward
T 1 206 622 2211
F 1 206 622 0308
W www.heffnermgmt.com
E marshaw@heffnermgmt.com

John Robert Powers
720 Olive Way, Suite 920
Seattle, WA 98101 USA
T 1 206 903 6900
F 1 206 903 0302

Kim Brooke Model/Talent Management
2044 Eastlake Avenue E
Seattle, WA 98102 USA
T 1 206 329 1111
F 1 206 328 5177

SEATTLE MODELS GUILD
1809 7th Avenue, Suite 608
Seattle, WA 98101 USA
Contact: Kristy Meyers
T 1 206 622 1406
F 1 206 622 8276
E kristy@smgmodels.com

TCM MODELS & TALENT
2200 6th Avenue, Suite 530
Seattle, WA 98121 USA
Contact: Terri Morgan, Owner
T 1 206 728 4826
F 1 206 728 1814
W www.tcmmodels.com
E terrim@www.tcmmodels.com

Team International
3431 96th Avenue NE
Seattle, WA 98004 USA
T 1 206 455 2969
F 1 206 455 2895

WHAT'S NEW, INC. GLOBAL ENTERTAINMENT NETWORK
1424 4th Avenue, 4th Floor
Seattle, WA 98101 USA
Contact: Marina Furuta
T 1 206 467 4972
F 1 206 467 4976
W www.whatsnewinc.com
E director@whatsnewinc.com

• • • • • • • • • •

DREZDEN INTERNATIONAL MODELING AGENCY & SCHOOL
3121 N Division Street
Spokane, WA 99207 USA
Contact: Patty or Walt Cromeenes
T 1 509 326 6800
F 1 509 327 0414
E drezdenmodels@hotmail.com

P.S.M. MODELS
PROFESSIONAL SCHOOL OF MODELING INC
18 N 59th Avenue
Yakima, WA 98908 USA
Contact: Penny Welch
T 1 509 965 1151
F 1 509 965 1151*51
E psmmodel@wolfnet.com

MODEL & TALENT AGENCIES

WISCONSIN

FIRST CHOICE TALENT & MODELING AGENCY INC
1718 Velp Avenue, Suite E
Green Bay, WI 54303 USA
Contact: Beverly Bodart, President
T 1 920 497 9609
F 1 920 497 9658
W www.firstchoicetalent.com
E info@firstchoicetalent.com

DYLAN SCOTT TALENT & MODEL CASTING
P.O. Box 44311
Madison, WI 53744-4311 USA
Contact: Theresa Boyeson
T 1 608 829 3739
F 1 608 827 9609
W www.dylanscott.com

THE ROCK AGENCY
2702 Monroe Street
Madison, WI 53711 USA
Contact: Raquel Repka
T 1 608 238 6372
F 1 608 238 6325
W www.modelingandtalent.com/rock/
E raquel@mailbag.com

Arlene Wilson Model Management
807 N Jefferson
Milwaukee, WI 53202 USA
T 1 414 283 5600
F 1 414 283 5610

JENNIFER'S TALENT UNLTD
740 N Plankinton Avenue, Suite 300
Milwaukee, WI 53203 USA
Contact: Jennifer Berg, President
T 1 414 277 9440
F 1 414 277 0918
W www.jenniferstalent.com
E jstalent@execpc.com

INTERNATIONAL AGENCIES

MODEL & TALENT AGENCIES

ARGENTINA • COUNTRY CODE: 54

DOTTO MODELS
Arenales 1938, Piso 4, Departamento B
Buenos Aires, 1124 Argentina
Contact: Pancho Dotto / Jorge E. Ruiz
T 11 4 814 0887
F 11 4 814 3626
W www.dottomodels.com.ar
E dottomod@infovia.com.ar

MODEL & TALENT AGENCIES

AUSTRALIA • COUNTRY CODE: 64

RACHEL'S MODEL MANAGEMENT & TRAINING
Quantas House, 144 North Terrace
Adelaide, SA 5000 Australia
Contact: Rachel Sanderson, Manager
T 8 8361 8113
F 8 8361 8132
W www.rachels.com.au
E rachel@rachels.com.au

Lisa Mann Creative Management
P.O. Box 1192
Bondi Junction, NS 1355 Australia
T 2 9387 8207
F 2 9389 0615

Brisbane

CL Agencies
32 O'Keefe Street, Woolloongabba
Brisbane, 4102 QLD Australia
T 7 3391 7733
F 7 3391 7583

DALLYS MODEL MANAGEMENT
Level 3, 150 Edward Street
Brisbane, QLD 4000 Australia
T 7 3221 1183
F 7 3221 3943
E dallys-model@management.tm

Lucas Theatrical Management
3-9 Metro Arts, 109 Edward Street
Brisbane, QLD 4000 Australia
T 7 3211 4345
F 7 3221 9191

TAMBLYN MODELS
Concorde House - Level 2, 217 George Street
Brisbane, Qld 4000 Australia
Contact: Sallie Tamblyn
T 7 3229 1299
F 7 3229 1243
E tamblyn@models.tm

Vivien's Model Management
Suite 1201, Level 12, MLC Centre, 239 George Street
Brisbane, QLD 4000 Australia
T 7 3221 2649
F 7 3220 0216

PARADOX MANAGEMENT
Suite 2, 193 Pacific Highway
Charlestown, NSW 2290 Australia
Contact: Samuel Saklaoui
T 2 4942 4911
F 2 4942 4870
W www.paradox.com.au
E paradox@paradoxm.com.au

BAYSIDE CHILDREN`S MODELLING AGENCY
10A Station Road, Suite 1
Cheltenham, VIC 3192 Australia
Contact: Marita Daniell, Director
T 3 9585 3422
F 3 9585 3844
W www.baysidebubs.management.tm
E baysidebubs@management.tm

EXPOSURE • THE AGENCY
FOR MODELS ACTORS EXTRAS
P.O. Box 711
Cronulla, NSW 2230 Australia
T 2 9181 2331
F 2 9719 2070

June Reilly Management
45 Cross Street Level 2
Double Bay, NSW 2028 Australia
T 2 9362 4604
F 2 9362 4765

Barry Michael Artists
14a Nelson Street
East St Kilda, VIC 3182 Australia
T 3 9534 2288
F 3 9525 3664

Genesis Model Management
P.O. Box 243
Fitzroy, VIC 3065 Australia
T 3 9416 2979
F 3 9416 0966

BODY IMPACT MODEL & TALENT AGENCY
79 Ryrie Street
Geelong, VIC 3220 Australia
Contact: Sharon Burgess, Director
T 500 527 528
T 352 233 242
F 352 233 242
E bodyimpact@ozemail.com.au

Penny Williams Management
181 Glebe Point Road, Level 2
Glebe, NSW 2037 Australia
T 2 9552 1701
F 2 9660 0434

Unique Models Agency
80 Rawson Road, P.O. Box 491
Greenacre, NS 2190 Australia
T 2 9708 5379
F 2 9785 7979

Image Management
Suite 2-3, 215 Brisbane Road
Labrador, QLD 4215 Australia
T 7 5537 4027
F 7 5529 1076

Melbourne

Bartuccio Dance & Promotion Centre
40 Green Street, Studio 4, Prahran
Melbourne, VIC 3181 Australia
T 3 9529 4299
F 3 9510 8956

CAMERON'S MANAGEMENT PTY LTD
3/402 Chapel Street, South Yarra, Suite 5
Melbourne, VIC 3134 Australia
Contact: Melinda Collette, Manager
T 3 9827 1687
F 3 9827 6401
W www.camerons.management.tm
E camerons-melb@management.tm

COSMOPOLITAN MODEL MANAGEMENT
537 Malvern Road, Toorak
Melbourne, VIC 3142 Australia
Contact: Deborah Miller
T 3 9823 1438
F 3 9826 5196
W www.cosmopolitan.management.tm
E cosmopolitan@management.tm

Elly Lukas Management
171 Collins Street
Melbourne, VIC 3000 Australia
T 3 9654 7777
F 3 9650 6777

HELENE ABICAIR MODEL & TALENT AGENCY
Level 2, Cenreway, 259 Collins Street
Melbourne, 3000 Australia
Contact: Helene Abicair, Director
T 3 9654 2037
F 3 9650 3192
E hrapl@02email.com.au

Jill's Casting Agency
6 Burston Road, Boronia
Melbourne, VIC 31SS Australia
T 3 9762 5328
F 3 9762 8724

Vivien's Model Management
209 Toorak Road, Suite 401, South Yarra
Melbourne, VIC 3141 Australia
T 3 9827 3155
F 3 9824 0074

• • • • • • • • • •

MODELS & ACTORS TALENT MANAGEMENT
98 Laman Street, Cooks Hill
Newcastle, NSW 2300 Australia
Contact: Trish Hanrahan
T 2 4927 0670
F 2 4927 0911
W www.modelsactorstm.com.au
E matm@idlnet.au

Perth

CARBERRY MODEL MANAGEMENT
Level 2, 90 King Street
Perth, WA 6000 Australia
Contact: Liz Carberry
Anthony Harden, Director
Tanya Muia, Booking Agent
T 8 9486 9994
F 8 9486 9995
E carberrymodels@primus.com.au

JEMMA INTERNATIONAL PTY LTD
Level 3, API House, 100 Murray Street
Perth, WA 6000 Australia
Contact: Maxine Howell-Price, Director
T 8 9421 1770
F 8 9421 1797
W www.jemma.com.au
E jemma@wantree.com.au

SPIERS MODEL MANAGEMENT
858 Hay Street
Perth, WA 6000 Australia
T 8 9322 1044
F 8 9322 1066
W www.spiersmodels.com
E spiers@wantree.com.au

TOP MODELS INTERNATIONAL
1st Floor, 158 William Street
Perth, WA 6000 Australia
T 8 9321 1339
F 8 9321 1209
W www.topmodels.com.au
E mail@topmodels.com.au

>>

AUSTRALIA

Prahran

Active Artists Management
1 High Street, 1st Floor
Prahran, VIC 3181 Australia
T 3 9521 2662
F 3 9521 1126

C.A.M. • China Arts Model Management
162 High Street
Prahran, VIC 3181 Australia
T 3 9525 1288
F 3 9521 3033

CHADWICK MODEL MANAGEMENT
31 Izzett Street, Suite 3
Prahran, VIC 3181 Australia
Contact: Matthew Anderson
T 3 9529 2177
F 3 9529 2178
W www.chadwick.management.tm
E chadwick-melb@management.tm

FRM MODEL MANAGEMENT
7, 2-22 Clifton Street
Prahran, VIC 3181 Australia
T 3 9521 5466
F 3 9521 4375
W www.frm.com.au
E mandi@ozemail.com.au

JM Agency
143A Chapel Street
Prahran, VIC 3181 Australia
T 3 9530 2150
F 3 9530 2151

• • • • • • • • • •

Cover Model International West Australia
P.O. Box 737
Scarborough, WA 6019 Australia
T 8 9445 7221
F 8 9446 2253

LOOKS & MODELS MANAGEMENT
41 Nerang Street
Southport, QLD 4215 Australia
Contact: Robert Veitch, Manager
T 7 5591 3581
F 7 5591 2852

Studio Search
Levell/4 Pinter Drive
Southport, QLD 4215 Australia
T 7 5531 1322
F 7 5531 1344

Epic Talent Management
15 Darling Street, P.O. Box 580
South Yarra, VIC 3141 Australia
T 3 9866 6386
F 3 9866 6389

GIANT MANAGEMENT PTY LTD
15 Darling Street, PO Box 580
South Yarra, VIC 3141 Australia
Contact: Greg Tyshing, President
T 3 9866 6455
F 3 9866 6389
W www.giant.management.tm
E giant@management.tm

Munchkins Management Pty Ltd
15 Darling Street, P.O. Box 626
South Yarra, VIC 3141 Australia
T 3 9821 5990
F 3 9821 5991

Kate's Kids
14a Nelson Street
St Kilda East, VIC 3182 Australia
T 3 9534 2288
F 3 9525 3664

LINDA'S INTERNATIONAL MANAGEMENT
12 Marine Pde, Suite 7D
St Kilda Beach, VIC 3182 Australia
Contact: Linda Ferguson, Director
T 3 9534 8755
F 3 9534 8566
E starmail@bigpond.net.au

FAYE ROLPH MODEL MANAGEMENT
3/7 Golf Street Maroochydore
Sunshine Coast, QLD 4558 Australia
Contact: Faye Rolph
T 7 5443 4522
F 7 5443 8685
E faye@faye-rolph-management.com

SCENE MODEL MANAGEMENT
Suite 201, 271 Cleveland Street
Surry Hills, NSW 2010 Australia
Contact: Vikki Graham, Director
Nev Stevenson, Head Booker
T 2 9318 2500
F 2 9318 2526
W www.scene.models.tm
E scene@models.tm

Sydney

ASAMI MODELS
Level 11, Elizabeth Towers
418A Elizabeth Street
Sydney, NSW Australia
Contact: Christopher Jones, Director
T 2 9282 6920
F 2 9282 6922
W http://asamimodels.com
E admin@asamimodels.com

CAMERON'S MANAGEMENT PTY LTD
2 New McLean Street, Suite 5, Edgecliff
Sydney, NSW 2027 Australia
Contact: Robert Newbould, Manager
T 2 9362 0100
F 2 9363 3317
W www.camerons.management.tm
E camerons@cameronsmanagement.com.au

CHADWICK MODEL MANAGEMENT
162 Goulburn Street, Level 10
Sydney, NSW 2000 Australia
Contact: Joseph Tenni
T 2 9261 0795
F 2 9261 0797
W www.chadwick.management.tm
E chadwick@chadwickma.com.au

CHIC MODEL MANAGEMENT
44 Roslyn Gardens, Elizabeth Bay
Sydney, NSW 2011 Australia
Contact: Ursula Hufnagl
T 2 9326 9488
F 2 9326 9921
W www.chic.management.tm
E chic@management.tm

Commercial Faces
Level 1, 308 Oxford St, Woollahra -
Sydney, NSW 2025 Australia
T 2 9389 9199
F 2 9389 9989

FACE MODELS
204 Crown Street, Darlinghurst
Sydney, NSW 2010 Australia
Contact: Shelley Williams
T 2 9332 4511
F 2 9332 4711
E face@models.tm

Gordon Management Group
Level 8, 140 William Street
East Sydney, NSW 2011 Australia
T 2 9326 9244
F 2 9326 9896

John Robert Powers
Level 2, 50 Margaret Street
Sydney, NSW Australia
T 2 9299 2227

June Cann Management
73 Jersey Road, Woollahra
Sydney, NSW 2025 Australia
T 2 9362 4007
F 2 9327 8553

Kubler Auckland Management
36A Bay Street, Double Bay
Sydney, NSW 1306 Australia
T 2 9362 8700
F 2 9362 8711

LCM Model Management
6/127 York Street
Sydney, NSW 2000 Australia
T 2 9267 1344
F 2 9267 1867

Lollipops Childrens Model Management
308 Oxford St, Woollahra -
Sydney, NSW 2025 Australia
T 2 9389 9199
F 2 9389 9989

PAMELA'S MODEL MANAGEMENT
196 Military Road, Neutral Bay, Suite 2
Sydney, NSW 2089 Australia
T 2 9908 3022
F 2 9908 4947

PG's Agency
2nd Floor, 371A Pitt Street
Sydney, NSW 2000 Australia
T 2 9267 5706
F 2 9283 3378

PLATFORM MODEL MANAGEMENT
Level 8, 140 William Street
East Sydney, NSW 2011 Australia
Contact: Georgia Douglas
T 2 9326 9711
F 2 9326 9896
W www.platform.models.tm
E platform@models.tm

PRISCILLA'S MODEL MANAGEMENT
204 Glenmore Road, Paddington
Sydney, NSW 2021 Australia
Contact: Priscilla Leighton Clark
T 2 9332 2422
F 2 9332 2488
W www.modelsonthenet.com.au
E priscillas@modelsonthenet.com.au

>>

AUSTRALIA

REGINES AGENCY / ICE MANAGEMENT
262 Pitt Street
Sydney, NSW 2000 Australia
Contact: Priscilla Leighton Clark
T 2 9267 2557
F 2 9267 2558
W www.sydney2000model.com
E regines@sydney2000model.com
E ice@sydney2000model.com

SHELLEY'S MODEL MANAGEMENT
204 Crown Street, Darlinghurst
Sydney, NSW 2010 Australia
Contact: Shelley Williams
T 2 9332 3755
F 2 9332 3855
E shelleys@management.tm

Spectrum Talent Mgmt
Spectrum Junior Models
Suite 4-154 Marsden Street, Parramatia
Sydney, NSW 2150 Australia
T 2 9635 6800
F 2 9635 1655

TMG • THE MODEL GENERATION
SPECTRUM TALENT MANAGEMENT
17 Langley Street, Darlinghurst
Sydney, NSW 2020 Australia
Contact: Michael Spott
T 2 9332 1777
F 2 9380 7530
W www.spectrum-tmg.management.tm
E spectrum-tmg@management.tm

Vivien's Model Management
43 Bay Street, Double Bay
Sydney, NSW 2028 Australia
T 2 9326 2700
F 2 9327 8084

• • • • • • • • • •

Team Agencies Pty Ltd
170 Kooyong Rd
Toorak, VIC 3142 Australia
T 3 9824 8877
F 3 9824 7666

FRM Management
621 Coronation Drive, Suite 3
Toowong, Australia
T 7 3871 0906
F 7 3871 1822

Kevin Palmer Management
258 Bulwara Road
Ultimo, NSW 2007 Australia
T 2 9552 1277
F 2 9660 3121

BARDOT'S BODIES
Suite 508, 63 Crown Street
Woolloomooloo, NSW 2011 Australia
Contact: Bessie Bardot
T 3 9360 0734
F 3 9380 7943
W www.bardotsbodies.com.au
E bessie@bardotbodies.com.au

BITE MODELS
Suite 508, 63 Crown Street
Woolloomooloo, NSW 2011 Australia
Contact: Ivo Tettamanti
T 3 9361 6090
F 3 9380 7943
W www.bitemodels.com
E ivo@bitemodels.com

MODEL & TALENT AGENCIES

AUSTRIA • COUNTRY CODE: 43

Visage Model Management
Landstr 42/3
Linz, A-4020 Austria
T 732 777 049
F 732 777 049 74

Magic Models
Sendlweg 5A
Salzburg, 5020 Austria
T 66 282 8196
F 66 282 8196 4

Vienna

AMT - Actors Models Talents
Ledergasse 22/8
Vienna, 1080 Austria
T 1 409 5944
F 1 409 5944 44

FAME INTERNATIONAL
Mahlerstrasse 13
Vienna, 1010 Austria
Contact: Peter Huber
T 1 513 9344
F 1 513 9943
W www.fame.at
E models@fame.at

Flair
Nusswaldgasse 19
Vienna, 1190 Austria
T 1 369 8436
F 1 369 1395

LOOK MODEL MANAGEMENT GMBH
Passauer Platz 1
Vienna, 1010 Austria
T 1 533 5816
F 1 535 4255
W www.lookmodels.at
E booking@lookmodels.at

NEXT COMPANY MODEL MANAGEMENT
Werdertorgasse 12
Vienna, 1010 Austria
Contact: Wolfgang Lackner
T 1 535 9669
F 1 535 0443

STELLA MODELS & TALENTS
Kaunitzgasse 9/6
Vienna, 1060 Austria
Contact: Roberta Manganelli
T 1 586 9027
F 1 586 9030
W www.stellamodels.com
E mail@stellamodels.com

VANITY FAIR
Frankgasse 1/17
Vienna, 1090 Austria
T 1 408 4314
T 1 408 4119
F 1 408 7076
W www.vanityfair.at
E vanityfair@usa.net

Wiener Modellsekretariat
Rudolfsplatz 10
Vienna, 1010 Austria
T 1 533 2277
F 1 535 3267

• • • • • • • • • •

Visage Model Managment
Siebensterngasse 52
Wien, A-1070 Austria
T 1 523 7170
F 1 523 7170 50

MODEL & TALENT AGENCIES

BELGIUM • COUNTRY CODE: 32

Brussels

DOMINIQUE MODELS AGENCY
48, Rue de Stassart
Brussels, 1050 Belgium
Contact: Dominique Fache
T 2 289 1189
F 2 289 1180
W www.dominique-models.be
E info@dominique-models.be

Gee Models Agency
Rue Paul Emile Janson 26
Brussels, 1050 Belgium
T 2 649 7770
F 2 649 8855

Loona Models Agency
Ave Louise 150
Brussels, 1050 Belgium
T 2 649 6042
F 2 640 1240

N.V. MODELS OFFICE INC
Sint-Annastraat 34
Brussels, 1000 Belgium
Contact: Marie Lou Eggermont, Director
T 2 511 4141
F 2 514 2326
W www.modelsoffice.com
E marilou@modelsoffice.be

New Models Agency
69 rue de Hennin
Brussels, B-1050 Belgium
T 2 644 3222
F 2 644 3262

Starmania
20, Avenue des Celtes
Brussels, B-1040 Belgium
T 2 732 1797
F 2 732 3018

Steff Model Management
58 Avenue de Stalingrad
Brussels, 1000 Belgium
T 2 511 6910
F 2 511 7075

MODEL & TALENT AGENCIES

BRAZIL • COUNTRY CODE: 55

DIESEL MODEL MANAGEMENT
Miguel Tostes 647, Suite 203
Porto Alegre, RS 90430-061 Brazil
Contact: Quin Vatson, President
T 51 333 5862
F 51 330 7349
W www.dieselmodels.com.br
E dieselmodels@hotmail.com

Elite Rio de Janeiro
Av Ataulfo de Paiva 706 cj 202 Leblon
Rio de Janeiro, 22440 Brazil
T 21 511 3437
F 21 259 5047

>>

BRAZIL

São Paulo

FORD MODELS
Rua Fidencio Ramos, 195
Vila Olimpia
São Paulo, 04551-010 Brazil
T 11 3049 8833
F 11 3049 8834

L'Equipe
Rua Marina Cintra 57, Jardim Europa
São Paulo, 01446-060 Brazil
T 11 3064 2811
F 11 3064 2811

MEGA
Rua Franz Schubert 184, Jardim Europa
São Paulo, 04571 Brazil
T 11 816 7675
F 11 870 3219

MODEL'S PROMOTERS
Av Brig Faria Lima, 2523-Cj12
São Paulo, SP 01451-001 Brazil
Contact: Regina Murca
T 11 3814 2022
F 11 3813 8766
E modelpromoters@uol.com.br

NEXT MANAGEMENT • SAO PAULO
Rua Funchal 573 I Andar
São Paulo, 04551-060 Brazil
T 11 3846 5678
F 11 3849 7210
W www.nextmodelmanagement.com

Taxi Model Agency
Av São Gabriel 564, Itaim,
São Paulo, 01435-000 Brazil
T 11 887 9755
F 11 885 8286

U:MA • UNITY MODEL AGENCY
R. Anacetuba, 71
São Paulo, SP 04531-040 Brazil
Contact: Caico de Queiroz, Director
T 11 3079 2994
F 11 3079 5925
E unitymodelagency@ual.com.br

VEGUE MODEL AGENCY
Rua Canario No 1100/Moema
Sao Paulo, SP 04521-005 Brazil
Contact: Bruno Bomeny, Director
T 11 5092 9011
T 11 9649 7113
F 11 533 2143
W www.vegue.com.br
E comercial@vegue.com.br

MODEL & TALENT AGENCIES

BULGARIA • COUNTRY CODE: 359

Underground Fashion Agency
89B Liuben Karavelov Street
Sofia, 1000 Bulgaria
T 2 963 25 63
F 2 963 25 63

J-Models
65 W Gladston Str., Fl 3
Sofia, 1000 Bulgaria
T 2 981 48 98
F 2 980 12 65

MODEL & TALENT AGENCIES

CANADA, ALBERTA

Calgary

Features Model & Talent Agency
12 Medford Place SW
Calgary, AB T2V 2E8 Canada
T 1 403 240 4468
F 1 403 240 0451

IMAGES INTERNATIONAL MODEL MANAGEMENT LTD.
578 Point McKay Grove NW
Calgary, AB T3B 5C5 Canada
Contact: Patricia (Pat) Collins
T 1 403 283 6517
F 1 403 283 6596
W www.imagesmodels.com
E iimm@home.com

MAG Models
Box 6, Site 9, RR #1
Calgary, AB T2P 2G4 Canada
T 1 403 541 0189
F 1 403 541 0189

Mode Models
#400, 933 17 Avenue SW
Calgary, AB T2T 5R6 Canada
T 1 403 216 2770
F 1 403 216 2771

OAKES MODEL MANAGEMENT
3911 Trasimene Circle SW
Calgary, AB T3E 7J6 Canada
Contact: Mr. Chad Oakes, President
T 1 403 240 0444
F 1 403 240 3756
W www.oakesmodels.com
E chadoakes@aol.com

PATTI FALCONER INTERNATIONAL MODEL & TALENT AGENCY
2523 17th Avenue SW
Calgary, AB T3E 0A2 Canada
Contact: Patti Falconer
T 1 403 249 8222
F 1 403 246 8916

• • • • • • • • • •

Mode Models
10080 Jasper Avenue, Suite 1004
Edmonton, AB T5J 1V9 Canada
T 1 780 424 6633
F 1 780 424 0898

SELECT MODEL MANAGEMENT LTD
306 Edmonton Centre
Edmonton, AB T5J 4H5 Canada
Contact: Larry Moore, President
T 1 780 482 2828
F 1 780 482 7605
W www.selectmodels.net
E select@compusmart.ab.ca

MODEL & TALENT AGENCIES

CANADA, BRITISH COLUMBIA

BBX MODEL & TALENT MANAGEMENT
10-1304 Ellis Street
Kelowna, BC V1Y 1Z8 Canada
Contact: Sylvia Fay, Owner/Director
T 1 250 762 7730
F 1 250 762 7741
E bbxmodels@home.com

LORI ALLAN INTERNATIONAL MODELS
1470 St Paul Street, Suite 204
Kelowna, BC VIY 2E6 Canada
Contact: Chris & Lori McCormack, Owners/Directors
T 1 250 861 5262
F 1 250 860 2030
T 1 250 491 1407

SPOTLIGHT ACADEMY FOR ACTORS & MODELS
2088 Sara's Way
Nanaimo, BC V9X 1K6 Canada
Contact: Jacqui Kaese
T 1 250 755 8975
F 1 250 722 2383
W www.spotlightacademy.com
E spotlight@home.com

LA MODE MODELING & TALENT AGENCY INC
Suite 201-1389 3rd Avenue
Prince George, BC V2L 3E8 Canada
Contact: Carolyn Sadler
T 1 250 561 2589
C 1 250 613 7906
F 1 250 561 2512
W www.lamodemodel.com
E carolyn@lamodemodel.com
*See Ad This Section.

LLOYD TALENT
14914-104 Avenue, Suite 106
Surrey, BC V3R 1M7 Canada
Contact: Lissa Lloyd / Chelsea Jamison
T 1 604 589 7559
F 1 604 658 3158
E lloyd@canadafilm.com

LMI • LISSA MODELS INTERNATIONAL
14914-104 Avenue, Suite 106
Surrey, BC V3R 1M7 Canada
Contact: Lissa Lloyd / Tom Gusway
T 1 604 589 7533
F 1 604 608 3158
W www.modelmgmt.com
E lmi@modelmgmt.com

>>

Vancouver

BLANCHE'S MODEL & TALENT MANAGEMENT
555 West 12th Avenue, Suite 100
Vancouver, BC V5Z 3X7 Canada
Contact: Melanie Hawthorne, Agency Director
T 1 604 685 0347
F 1 604 669 1415
E blanches@blanchemacdonald.com

CHARLES STUART INTERNATIONAL MODELS
314-1008 Homer Street
Vancouver, BC V6B 2X1 Canada
Contact: Charles Stuart, President
T 1 604 222 3177
F 1 604 228 4039
W www.faceswest.com
E charlesstuart@telus.net

FORD MODELS
Suite 206-1118 Homer Street
Vancouver, BC V6B 6L5 Canada
T 1 604 899 0456
F 1 604 899 8987

JOHN CASABLANCAS VANCOUVER MODEL MANAGEMENT
220 Cambie Street, Suite 150
Vancouver, BC V6B 2M9 Canada
Contact: Lori & James Falconer
T 1 604 688 0261
F 1 604 688 4229
W www.vancouvertalent.com
E info@vancouvertalent.com

LIZBELL AGENCY LTD
304-1228 Hamilton Street
Vancouver, BC V6B 2S8 Canada
Contact: Liz Bell, Owner
T 1 604 683 9696
F 1 604 683 3414
W www.lizbellagency.com
E lizbell@axionet.com

Look Management
110-1529 W 6th Avenue
Vancouver, BC V6J 1R1 Canada
T 1 604 737 5225
F 1 604 737 7612

PT MODELS SCOUTING INC
7431 McCallen Road, Richmond
Vancouver, BC V7C 2H6 Canada
Contact: Jill Sheu, Managing Director
T 1 604 272 6605
F 1 604 272 6605
E ptmodels@kimo.com.tw

RICHARD'S INTERNATIONAL MODEL MANAGEMENT
Hotel Vancouver, 900 West Georgia Street, Suite 103
Vancouver, BC V6C 2W6 Canada
Contact: Richard, Robbin or Gerry
T 1 604 683 7484
F 1 604 683 7485
E richardmodels@hotmail.com

TOP MODELS INC / BELLA MODELS
615-1033 Davie Street
Vancouver, BC V6E 1M7 Canada
Contact: Sonya Siltani
T 1 604 844 7808
F 1 604 844 7807
E bella-models@hotmail.com

Vanity Management Inc
400-601 W Broadway
Vancouver, BC V5Z 4C2 Canada
T 1 604 675 6962
F 1 604 675 6984

VMH INTERNATIONAL MODELS
1311 Howe Street, Suite 200
Vancouver, BC V6Z 2P3 Canada
Contact: Vanessa M. Helmer
T 1 604 221 4080
F 1 604 221 4071
W www.vmhmodels.com
E info@vmhmodels.com

• • • • • • • • • •

BARBARA COULTISH TALENT & MODEL MANAGEMENT
101A-2526 Government Street
Victoria, BC V8T 4P7 Canada
Contact: Barbara Coultish, Talent Division
or Laura Coultish, Model Division
T 1 250 382 2670
F 1 250 382 2691
E bcoultish@telus.net

Bonnie Pollard's Fashion in Motion
3542 Blanshard Street, Suite 201
Victoria, BC V8X 1W3 Canada
T 1 250 475 3355
F 1 250 475 4434

JÄGER MODEL & TALENT MANAGEMENT
P.O. Box 5712, Station B
Victoria, BC V8R 6S8 Canada
Contact: Gail Smith
T 1 250 595 0420
F 1 250 595 0480
E jagermodels@hotmail.com

MODEL & TALENT AGENCIES

CANADA, MANITOBA

BDM Talent Inc
P.O. Box 35031, Henderson RPO
Winnipeg, MB R2K 4J9 Canada
T 1 204 488 9343
F 1 204 667 5705

PANACHE MODEL & TALENT MANAGEMENT
106-897 Corydon Avenue
Winnipeg, MB R3M 0W7 Canada
Contact: Jane Campbell
T 1 204 982 6150
F 1 204 474 2687
W www.panacheagency.mb.ca
E panache@pangea.ca

MODEL & TALENT AGENCIES

CANADA, NEW BRUNSWICK

Ruth Barnes Modeling Agency Ltd
585 Mountain Road
Moncton, NB E1C 2N9 Canada
T 1 506 854 3318
F 1 506 383 9273

MODEL & TALENT AGENCIES

CANADA, NEWFOUNDLAND

X-POSURE INTERNATIONAL INC
21 Hyde Park Drive
St John's, NFLD A1A 5G1 Canada
Contact: Ms. Alma Connock
T 1 709 579 2996
F 1 709 726 3956
W www.x-posuremodels.com
E x-posure.models@roadrunner.nf.net

MODEL & TALENT AGENCIES

CANADA, NOVA SCOTIA

CITY MODELS • MODEL & TALENT AGENCY
6436 Quinpool Road, 2nd Floor
Halifax, NS B3L 1B1 Canada
Contact: Carol Iannuzzi, Director
T 1 902 422 1444
T 1 902 462 1047
F 1 902 462 2574

The Cassidy Group
5212 Sackville Street, Suite 200
Halifax, NS B3J 1K6 Canada
T 1 902 492 4410
F 1 902 492 4411

MODEL & TALENT AGENCIES

CANADA, ONTARIO

INTERNATIONAL MODEL MANAGEMENT
25 Dunlop Street East
Barrie, ON L4M 5A1 Canada
Contact: Christine Grigor, New Faces Director
T 1 705 739 8285
F 1 705 739 7024
W www.michelesintl.com
E info@michelesintl.com

Potentials
28 Stoney Brook Center
Barrie, ON L4N 0A5 Canada
T 1 705 722 5410
F 1 705 722 3233

Mode Elle
291 Front Street
Belleville, ON K8N 2Z6 Canada
T 1 613 967 0470
F 1 613 967 1544

Lydia's International Children Modeling Agency
3280 Mead Crescent
Burlington, ON L7M 3M2 Canada
T 1 905 336 9164
F 1 905 315 8589

Latin Talent Agency
2035 Highway Seven W
Concord, ON L4K 1V6 Canada
T 1 905 738 5323
F 1 905 738 4679

ANGIE'S MODELS & TALENT INC
4 Second Street East
Cornwall, ON K6H 1Y3 Canada
Contact: Angie & Lou Seymour
T 1 613 932 1451
F 1 613 933 5537
W www.angiesmodels.com
E angies@canadafilm.com
***See Ad This Section.**

Vogue Models & Talent
36 Hess Street, S 3rd Floor
Hamilton, ON L8P 3N1 Canada
T 1 905 523 5077
F 1 905 529 9616

Merit Model Management
1097 Frost Drive
Kingston, ON K7M 5N4 Canada
T 1 613 634 4140
F 1 613 634 7420

>>

NV • New Vision Models
303 Bagot Street, La Salle Mews, Suite 1, Box 23
Kingston, ON K7K 5W7 Canada
T 1 613 544 2200
F 1 613 544 8276

Towne Models
1160 Clyde Court
Kingston, ON K7P 2E4 Canada
T 1 613 384 5223
F 1 613 384 8601

THE GEMINI GROUP
127 Weber Street East
Kitchener, ON N2H 4A1 Canada
Contact: Audrey Wilson, Models Division
or Jessie Winkler, Talent Division
T 519 578 2111
F 1 519 578 2226
W www.geminimodels.com
E audrey@geminimodels.com

Elegance
219 Oxford Street W, Suite 302
London, ON N6H 1S5 Canada
T 1 519 434 1181
F 1 519 434 1182

NOW MODELLING & ACTING
575 Richmond St, 2nd Floor
London, ON N6A 3G2 Canada
Contact: Jennifer Orlebar, Agency Director
A Full Service Model & Talent Agency
Modelling • Acting • Self Improvement • Fashion Shows • Corporate Image
T 1 519 432 1161
F 1 519 432 1229

Barbizon
1590 Dundas Street E, Suite 208
Mississauga, ON L4X 2Z2 Canada
T 1 905 949 5151
F 1 905 949 2748

ZAIDI MODELS
50 Burnhamthorpe Road West, Suite 348
Mississauga, ON L5B 3C2 Canada
Contact: Hassain Zaidi, Agency Director
T 1 905 803 9040
F 1 905 803 9043
W www.zaidimodels.com
E contact@zaidimodels.com
***See Ad This Section.**

FMI • Flare Modeling Inc/Flare Talent
444 Timothy Street
Newmarket, ON L3Y 1P8 Canada
T 1 905 898 1149
F 1 905 898 1147

GEOFFERY CHAPMAN MODELS
6153 Main Street
Niagara Falls, ON L2G 6A3 Canada
Contact: Geoffrey Chapman
T 1 905 374 3821
F 1 905 374 1134
W www.geoffreychapman.com
E geoff@geoffreychapman.com

Farmer's Modeling School & Agency
P.O. Box 369
Ohsweken, ON N0A 1M0 Canada
T 1 519 445 2851
F 1 519 445 4995

ANGIE'S MODELS & TALENT INC
25A York Street
Ottawa, ON K1N 5S7 Canada
Contact: Angie & Lou Seymour
T 1 613 244 0544
F 1 613 244 0481
W www.angiesmodels.com
E angies@canadafilm.com
***See Ad This Section.**

BARRETT PALMER MODELS INTERNATIONAL INC
410 Queen Street, 1st Floor
Ottawa, ON K1R 5A7 Canada
T 1 613 235 5145
F 1 613 235 0213
E bpmodels@netcom.ca

MODELS INTERNATIONAL MANAGEMENT
185 Somerset Street W, Suite 312
Ottawa, ON K2P 0J2 Canada
Contact: Julie Pellerin, President
T 1 613 236 9575
F 1 613 236 9607
W www.modelsinternational.on.ca
E modelsintmgmt@primus.ca

Lasting Beauty Model Management
1330 Pembroke Street West, Unit 14
Pembroke, ON K8A 7A3 Canada
T 1 613 732 0098
F 1 613 735 4324

L'Image Model Management
93 Pilgrim Street
Sault Ste Marie, ON P6A 3E6 Canada
T 1 705 945 6144
F 1 705 942 9335

Gloria Moody Models/Agcy
522 Piper Avenue
Thunder Bay, ON P7E 4T5 Canada
T 1 807 622 9084
F 1 807 626 8270

Lakehead Modeling School
176 Rupert Street
Thunder Bay, ON P7B 3X1 Canada
T 1 807 344 5973
F 1 807 346 0915

Toronto

ACI Talent
401 Richmond Street W, Suite 401
Toronto, ON M5V 3A8 Canada
T 1 416 408 3304
F 1 416 408 4867

APPLAUSE / BICKERTON MODEL & TALENT
499 Main Street South, Suite 208
Toronto, ON L6Y 1N7 Canada
Contact: Favra or Eddi
T 1 905 457 7571
F 1 905 457 3048

ARMSTRONG INTERNATIONAL
78 Berkeley Street
Toronto, ON M5A 2W7 Canada
T 1 416 594 0455
T 1 800 618 2825 Toll Free
T 1 416 594 9820 Men
T 1 416 594 9835 Women
T 1 416 594 9848 Kool Kids
T 1 416 594 0533 TV/Film
F 1 416 594 9926
W www.armstrongmodels.com
E information@armstrongmodels.com

B & M MODEL MANAGEMENT
645 King Street West, Suite 401
Toronto, ON M5V 1M5 Canada
Contact: Brooke Bailey / Mel Mateus
T 1 416 925 8722
F 1 416 925 1277
E info@bnmmodels.com

Blast! Models Inc
615 Yonge Street, Suite 200
Toronto, ON M4Y 1Z5 Canada
T 1 416 922 7205
F 1 416 922 1874

Broadbelt & Fonte Models Inc
696 Dufferin Street
Toronto, ON M6K 2B5 Canada
T 1 416 588 8806
F 1 416 588 4984

Butler Ruston Bell Talent Associates Inc
10 St Mary Street, Suite 308
Toronto, ON M4Y 1P9 Canada
T 1 416 964 6660
F 1 416 960 8979

Characters Talent
150 Carlton
Toronto, ON M5A 2K1 Canada
T 1 416 964 8522
F 1 416 964 6349

CAROLYN'S MODEL & TALENT AGENCY
STUDIO TALENT MANAGEMENT
2104 Yonge Street
Toronto, ON M4S 2A5 Canada
Contact: Carolyn Nikkanen
T 1 416 544 0232
F 1 416 544 1948

Christopher Banks & Associates
6 Adelaide Street E, Suite 610
Toronto, ON M5C 1H6 Canada
T 1 416 214 1155
F 1 416 214 1150

Delio Talent Agency
1357 Bathurst Street, 3rd Floor
Toronto, ON M5R 3H8 Canada
T 1 416 928 9197
F 1 416 928 9121

>>

DISTINCT LOOK AGENCY
783 Lawrence Avenue W, Suite 12B
Toronto, ON M6A 1C2 Canada
Contact: Volda Alexander, Talent Director
T 1 416 787 6423
F 1 416 787 2034

ELEANOR FULCHER INTERNATIONAL
615 Yonge Street, Suite 200
Toronto, ON M4Y 1Z5 Canada
Contact: Clarissa Siebert, Agency Director
T 1 416 922 1945
F 1 416 922 1874
W www.eleanorfulcher.com
E efagency@interlog.com

Elite Models
477 Richmond Street W, Suite 301
Toronto, ON M5V 3E7 Canada
T 1 416 369 9995
F 1 416 369 1929

EMMERSON DENNEY PERSONAL MANAGEMENT
119 Portland Street
Toronto, ON M5V 2N4 Canada
T 1 416 504 9666
F 1 416 504 7454

FORD CANADA
385 Adelaide St W, 2nd Floor
Toronto, ON M5V 1S4 Canada
Contact: Cynthia Cully
Contact: Jeff Andrews for Talent
Contact: Pamela McLean for Just 4 Kids
T 1 416 362 9208
T 1 416 362 7273 Talent
T 1 416 362 8344 Just 4 Kids
F 1 416 362 9604
E ford@canadafilm.com

Gary Goddard & Associates
10 St Mary Street, Suite 305
Toronto, ON M4Y 1P9 Canada
T 1 416 928 0299
F 1 416 924 9593

Hollywood North Inc
18 Thurston Road
Toronto, ON M4S 2V7 Canada
T 1 416 481 1000
F 1 416 486 5500

ICE MODEL MANAGEMENT
165 Bathurst Street, 1st Floor
Toronto, ON M5V 3C2 Canada
T 1 416 366 7890
F 1 416 203 6267
W www.icemodels.com
E melora@icemodels.com

Jack Frizelle Talent
1357 Bathurst Street, 3rd Floor
Toronto, ON M5R 3H8 Canada
T 1 416 530 0550
F 1 416 928 9121

Jack Timlock
402 Sherbourne Street, Suite 2
Toronto, ON M4X 1K3 Canada
T 1 416 923 1914
F 1 416 923 3757

Jordan & Assoc Talent Management
615 Yonge Street, Suite 401
Toronto, ON M4Y 1Z5 Canada
T 1 416 515 2028
F 1 416 515 1763

Joy Davies Agency
P.O. Box 699, Postal Station F
Toronto, ON M4Y 2N6 Canada
T 1 416 410 2414

JUST MODELS INC
901 Yonge Street, Suite 200
Toronto, ON M4W 3M2 Canada
Contact: Marinos Dafnas, Owner
T 1 416 961 7888
F 1 416 961 8788
W www.justmodelsinc.com
E jumodels@idirect.com

KG Talent
55 A Sumach
Toronto, ON M5A 3J6 Canada
T 1 416 368 4866
F 1 416 368 2492

Lorraine Wells & Co
10 St Mary Street, Suite 320
Toronto, ON M4Y 1P9 Canada
T 1 416 413 1676
F 1 416 413 1680

McGuin & Assoc Inc
10 St Mary Street, Suite 307
Toronto, ON M4Y 1P9 Canada
T 1 416 920 6884
F 1 416 920 8543

Messinger Agency
The Colonnade, 131 Bloor Street W, Suite 515-G
Toronto, ON M5S 1R1 Canada
T 1 416 960 1000
F 1 416 960 1001

Newton Landry Management Inc
19 Isabella Street
Toronto, ON M4Y 1M7 Canada
T 1 416 960 8683
F 1 416 960 6015

NEXT MANAGEMENT • TORONTO
110 Spadina Avenue, Suite 303
Toronto, ON M5V 2K4 Canada
T 1 416 603 4807
F 1 416 603 9891
W www.nextmodelmanagement.com
***See Ad This Section.**

Oscars Abrams & Zimel Inc
438 Queens Street E
Toronto, ON M5A 1T4 Canada
T 1 416 860 1790
F 1 416 860 0236

>>

PERRY D. ANDREWS TALENT MGMT (P.A.T.M)
PERRY D. ANDREWS MODEL MGMT
PERRY D. ANDREWS "NEW FACES"
599-B Yonge Street, Suite 342
Toronto, ON M4Y 1Z4 Canada
Contact: Perry Andrews, Kent Simmons, or Michelle Kay
T 1 416 961 2727
F 1 416 944 0946

Phoenix Artists Management
10 St Mary Street, Suite 810
Toronto, ON M4Y 1P9 Canada
T 1 416 964 6464
F 1 416 969 9924

Premier Artists Management
671 Danforth Avenue, Suite 305
Toronto, ON M4J 1L3 Canada
T 1 416 461 6868
F 1 416 461 7677

Reinhart/Perkins Inc
2120 Queen Street East, Suite 300
Toronto, ON M4E 1E2 Canada
T 1 416 699 7130
F 1 416 699 1101

SHERRIDA PERSONAL MANAGEMENT INC
110 Scollard Street
Toronto, ON M5R 1G2 Canada
Contact: Sherrida Rawlings / Rebecca Rawlings
T 1 416 928 2323
F 1 416 928 0767
E mgmt@sherrida.com

SUBZERO MODEL MANAGEMENT
624 Richmond Street W
Toronto, ON M5V 3C2 Canada
T 1 416 203 6522
F 1 416 203 6267
W www.subzeromodels.com
E szmm@subzeromodels.com

Sutherland Models Inc
174 Spadina Avenue
Toronto, ON M5T 2C2 Canada
T 1 416 703 7070
F 1 416 703 9726

Talent House
204 A St George Street
Toronto, ON M5R 2N6 Canada
T 1 416 960 9686
F 1 416 960 2314

Trainco Ltd
145 Highbore Road, Suite 1
Toronto, ON M5P 2J8 Canada
T 1 416 923 2884
F 1 416 923 1520

Worldwide Talent
20 Bay Street, Suite 1205
Toronto, ON M5J 2N8 Canada
T 1 416 410 6443
F 1 416 932 8910

ZAIDI MODELS
325 King Street West, Suite 202
Toronto, ON M5V 1J5 Canada
Contact: Hassain Zaidi, Agency Director
T 1 416 595 1010
F 1 416 595 9785
W www.zaidimodels.com
E contact@zaidimodels.com
***See Ad This Section.**

• • • • • • • • • • •

Cameo Models
51 Albert Street
Waterloo, ON N2L 3S1 Canada
T 1 519 885 0919
F 1 519 885 3435

HARLOW MODEL MANAGEMENT
101 Dundas Street W, 2nd Floor
Whitby, ON L1N 2M2 Canada
Contact: Viveca Rupa
T 1 905 430 5716
F 1 905 430 9366

LA MAGIQUE MODELLING AGENCIE & SCHOOL
5614 Wyandotte Street East
Windsor, ON N8S 1M3 Canada
Contact: Simona Gesuale / Kate Derbyshire
T 1 519 974 4441
F 1 519 974 4441
E magique@mnsi.net

MODEL & TALENT AGENCIES

CANADA, QUEBEC

Aviel Talent Management
5784 Westluke Avenue
Cote Saint Luc, QB H4W 2N7 Canada
T 1 514 481 9065
F 1 514 481 3879

Mannequins Cristal
136 de Gallichan
Gatineau, QB J8R 2Y4 Canada
T 1 819 663 0747
F 1 819 663 0747

Montreal

Agence Girafe
28 rue Notre Dame Est, Suite 302
Montreal, QB H2Y 1B9 Canada
T 1 514 866 1830
F 1 514 866 2939

AGENCE SCOOP
405 St-Jean Baptiste, Suite 2
Montreal, Quebec H2Y 2Z7 Canada
Contact: Jean-Philippe Collin & Sylvie Beaulac
T 1 514 875 6361
F 1 514 861 4885
E scoop@qc.aira.com

AGENCE SYBILLE SASSE
1600 Notre Dame St W, Suite 205
Montreal, QB H3J 1M1 Canada
Contact: Sybille Sasse
T 1 514 934 0393
F 1 514 934 0326
E sybillesasse@qc.aibn.com

Cosmos Modeling Agency
1134 rue Ste-Catherine Ouest, Suite 510
Montreal, QB H3B 1H4 Canada
T 1 514 908 2220
F 1 514 487 4673

FOCUS INTERNATIONAL
1134 rue Ste-Catherine Ouest, Suite 510
Montreal, QB H3B 1H4 Canada
Contact: Sergio Panzera, Owner
T 1 514 866 8846
F 1 514 866 8748
E focus@contact.net

Folio Montreal
295 rue de la Commune Ouest
Montreal, QB H2Y 2E1 Canada
T 1 514 288 8080
F 1 514 843 5597

GIOVANNI MODEL MANAGEMENT
291 Place d'Youville
Montreal, QB H2Y 2B5 Canada
Contact: Jean Francois
T 1 514 845 1278
F 1 514 845 2547
E montreal@giovannimodels.com

Giraffe Agency
28 Notre-Dame E, Suite 302
Montreal, QB H2Y 1B9 Canada
T 1 514 866 1830
F 1 514 866 2939

>>

CANADA, QUEBEC

Glenn Talent Management
3981 Street Laurent, Suite 600
Montreal, QB H2W 1Y5 Canada
T 1 514 499 3485
F 1 514 499 3491

John Casablancas/MTM
Galeries Dauphin Sud, 3535 Papineau, Suite 2804
Montreal, QB H2K 4J9 Canada
T 1 514 527 8484
F 1 514 527 9530

K.L. Benzakein Talent Inc
1445 Lambert Classe, 2nd Floor
Montreal, QB H3Y 2S4 Canada
T 1 514 931 9260
F 1 514 931 9246

Le Petit Monde Agency
179 rue Sherbrooke Est
Montreal, QB H2X 1C7 Canada
T 1 514 845 6495
F 1 514 845 6495

Lyne Lemleux Agency
5130 rue Saint Hubart, Suite 208
Montreal, QB H2J 2Y3 Canada
T 1 514 273 3411
F 1 514 495 9045

Micheline Saint Laurent Agency
10840 rue Saint Francois d'Assise
Montreal, QB H2B 2N5 Canada
T 1 514 383 8378
F 1 514 388 8178

Montage Inc
3451 Street Laurent, Suite 400
Montreal, QB H2X 2T6 Canada
T 1 514 284 4901
F 1 514 284 3656

NEXT MANAGEMENT • MONTREAL
3547 boul St Laurent, Suite 401
Montreal, QB H2X 2T6 Canada
T 1 514 288 9216
F 1 514 288 9043
W www.nextmodelmanagement.com
***See Ad This Section.**

Orlando Galletta Inc
6397 St Denis Street
Montreal, QB H2S 2R8 Canada
T 1 514 270 8236
F 1 514 278 8807

Payer et Choquet Agency
5298 boul Pie IX
Montreal, QB H1X 2B7 Canada
T 1 514 728 2811
F 1 514 728 1405

Premier Role Inc
3449 de l'Hotel de ville
Montreal, QB H2X 3B5 Canada
T 1 514 844 7653
F 1 514 848 9636

Specs
3981 Boulevard Street Laurent, Suite 710
Montreal, QB H2W 1Y5 Canada
T 1 514 844 1352
F 1 514 844 8540

• • • • • • • • • •

Duchesne Agency
30 av Marsolais, Suite 1
Outremont, QB H2V 1N2 Canada
T 1 514 274 4607
F 1 514 274 0591

Ginette Achim Agency
1053 Laurier
Outremont, QB H2V 2L2 Canada
T 1 514 271 3737
F 1 514 271 8774

Maxime Vanasse Agency
853 av Rockland
Outremont, QB H2V 2Z8 Canada
T 1 514 277 4842
F 1 514 277 4817

Nicole Dodier Agency
2 rue Saint Malo
Sainte Julie, QB J0L 2S0 Canada
T 1 450 649 4611
F 1 450 922 4461

MacDonald Cartier School
7445 Chemin Chambly
St Hubert, QB J3Y 3S3 Canada
T 1 450 678 1070
F 1 450 678 9335

Agence de Mannequin Bellini International
5099A Jarry Est
St Leonard, QB H1R 1Y5 Canada
T 1 514 326 3599
F 1 514 329 0281

MODEL & TALENT AGENCIES

CANADA, SASKATCHEWAN

Edge Models & Talent Agency
10 Odin Walk
Regina, SASK S4S 6W5 Canada
T 1 306 789 2403
F 1 306 586 2468

Stages Model Agency
#304-2206 Dewdney Avenue
Regina, SASK S4R 1H3 Canada
T 1 306 757 8370
F 1 306 522 2271

MG Model & Talent Management
208-1001 22nd Street W
Saskatoon, SASK S7M 0S2 Canada
T 1 306 653 3830
F 1 306 653 4916

She Modeling Agency & School
3211 Wells Avenue
Saskatoon, SASK S7K 5W4 Canada
T 1 306 652 7484
F 1 306 382 4513

MODEL & TALENT AGENCIES

CHILE • COUNTRY CODE: 56

Academia y Agencia de Modelos Ximena Caceres
1 Oriente 312
Vina del Mar, Chile
T 32 697 736
F 32 697 737

ELITE CHILE
Don Carlos 3269
Oficina 1, Las Condes
Santiago, Chile
Contact: Ofelia Memoli, Booker
T 2 334 7036
F 2 245 1345
W www.elitechile.cl
E elite@cmet.net

Gabriel Munoz Escuela de Modelos
Roman Diaz 55
Santiago, Chile
T 2 235 4903
F 2 236 0519

NEW MODELS AGENCY
Suecia 2788
Santiago, 6840137 Chile
Contact: Simone Lindeberg
T 2 341 3060
F 2 204 8810
E nwmodels@entelchile.net

MODEL & TALENT AGENCIES

CHINA • COUNTRY CODE: 86

Galaxy Model Management
3/F No 3 Dong Fang Road, Dong San Huan Bei Lu
Beijing, 100027 China
T 10 6462 8134
F 10 6462 8148

MODEL & TALENT AGENCIES

CROATIA • COUNTRY CODE: 385

Face Model Management
L. Milenica 31
Rijeka, 51000 Croatia
T 51 223 812
F 51 261 182

Zagreb

Look
Manzoni 2
Zagreb, 10000 Croatia
T 51 214 026
F 51 214 407

M.A.G.I.K & Oberon
Baboniceva 34
Zagreb, 10000 Croatia
T 1 463 5338
F 1 463 5338

MIDIKEN MODEL MANAGEMENT
Svarcova 18
Zagreb, 10000 Croatia
Contact: Hamed Bangoura / Daouda Bangoura
T 1 2303 730
T 1 2303 729
T 1 2312 695
F 1 2312 420
W www.midiken.hr
E mouhamed@midiken.hr

WWW MANAGEMENT
Radiceva 34
Zagreb, 10000 Croatia
Contact: Nedad Drk, President
T 1 492 1800
F 1 488 3333
W http://WWWManagement.net/models
E models@WWWManagement.net

MODEL & TALENT AGENCIES

CZECH REPUBLIC • COUNTRY CODE: 42

D.F.C. Fashion Club / Genage Models
Vesela 5 Street
Brno, 602 00 Czech Republic
T 6 0273 0104
F 5 4221 1718

DOM Production CZ Ltd
Novobranska 3
Brno, 602 00 Czech Republlic
T 5 4251 0105
F 5 4222 1943

Prague

ABSOLUT MODEL AGENCY
Katerinska 7
Prague 2, 12000 Czech Republic
Contact: Luda Antolikova
T 2 9621 0561
F 2 9621 0561
E luda@absolutmodel.cz

Bohemia Models
Jungmannova 24
Prague, 11000 Czech Republic
T 2 2494 7367
F 2 2494 6367

COMPANY MODELS
Drtinova 8
Prague 5, 150 00 Czech Republic
Contact: David Kominek, Managing Director
T 2 5701 8650
F 2 5701 8138
W www.companymodels.cz
E dkominek@yahoo.com

LOOK MODEL MANAGEMENT
Trziste 8
Prague 1, 1100 Czech Republic
T 2 57 53 14 22
T 00 381 63 387 783 Mobile
F 2 57 53 05 10
W www.lookmodels.cz
E lookmodel@volny.cz

Rhea Model Management
Machova 21
Prague 2, 12000 Czech Republic
T 2 2251 6955
F 2 2251 6955

Studio 91
Rasinovo Nabrezi 26
Prague 2, 12800 Czech Republic
T 2 290 405
F 2 290 604

MODEL & TALENT AGENCIES

DENMARK • COUNTRY CODE: 45

Diva Models
Guldsmedgade 22
Arhus C, 8000, Denmark
T 8619 7444
F 8612 5950

MODELBUREAUET MODELBOOKING APS
Frederiksgade 12-14
Arhus C, 8000 Denmark
Contact: Carlotte Hasse, Owner
T 8619 6888
F 8619 6388
W www.modelbooking.com
E mette@modelbooking.com

Copenhagen

2PM MODEL MANAGEMENT
Norregade 2, 1st Floor
Copenhagen, 1165 K Denmark
T 33 76 62 62
F 33 76 62 63
W www.2pm.dk
E 2pm@2pm.dk

BC Models
Kompagnistraede 21
Copenhagen k, 1208 Denmark
T 3313 0991
F 3313 0937

Best CPH Model Management
Studiestraede 24
Copenhagen, 1455 Denmark
T 3312 7177
F 3312 7078

BOOKING HOUSE
Ny Adelgade 8
Copenhagen, 1104 K Denmark
Contact: Nanna Berg, Manager
T 3337 0710
F 3333 0790
W www.bookinghouse.dk
E info@bookinghouse.dk

FLAIR MODELS
Hoejbroplads 3
Copenhagen, 1200 Denmark
Contact: Jesper Christiansen
T 7026 2644
F 7026 2655
W www.flair-models.dk
E info@flair-models.dk

SCANDINAVIAN MODELS / ELITE COPENHAGEN
Gothersgade 89, Ground Floor
Copenhagen, 1123 K Denmark
Contact: Trice Tomsen, Director
T 33 93 24 24
T 33 15 14 14
F 33 93 92 24
W www.scanelite.dk
E trice@scanelite.dk

Scoop Models of Copenhagen ApS
Læderstræde 9
Copenhagen K, DK-1201 Denmark
T 3314 1013
F 3314 1031

Unique Models
Ny Østergrade 3
Copenhagen K, 1107 Denmark
T 3312 0055
F 3312 0550

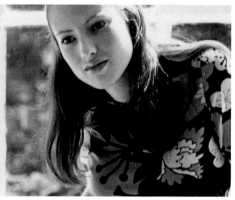

MODEL & TALENT AGENCIES

ECUADOR • COUNTRY CODE: 593

FINNEGAN GROUP
Quiteno Libre 117
Quito, Ecuador
Contact: David Finnegan
T 2 893 586
F 2 896 032
E dfinnega@uio.satnet.net

MODEL & TALENT AGENCIES

ENGLAND • COUNTRY CODE: 44

BMA Model Agency
The Stables, Norcott Hall Barns, Norcott Hill
Berkhamsted, Herts, HP4 IRB England
T 1442 878 878
F 1442 879 879

MOT Model Agency
The Stables, Ashlyns Hall, Chesham Road
Berkhamsted, Herts, HP4 2ST England
T 1 442 863 918
F 1 442 873 333

Adage Model Agency
The Custard Factory, Gibb Street
Birmingham, B9 4AA England
T 121 693 4040
F 121 693 4041

NEMESIS
95 Spencer Street, The Jewelry Quarter
Birmingham, B18 6DA England
Contact: Nigel Martin-Smith, Managing Director
T 121 554 7878
F 121 554 6526
W www.nemesisagency.co.uk
E jo@nmsmanagement.co.uk

United Colours of London Ltd
1 Penylan Place
Edgeware, Middlesex, HA8 6EN England
T 208 952 2941
F 208 952 1892

Elisabeth Smith Ltd
81 Headstone Road
Harrow, Middlesex, HA1 1PQ England
T 208 863 2331
F 208 861 1880

Scallywags
1 Cranbrook Rise,
Ilford, Essex, IG1 3QW England
T 208 518 1133
F 208 924 0262

Pat Keeling Model Agency
99-101 Highcross Street
Leicester, LE1 4PH England
T 116 262 2540
F 116 253 7712

London

ANGELS
52 Queens Gardens, Suite 6
London, W2 3AA England
Contact: Angela Papadopoulos
T 207 262 5344
F 207 402 2201
W www.angels-agency.com
E models@angels-agency.com

Assassin Management
2 Marshall Street
London, W1V 1LQ England
T 207 534 5400
F 207 534 5401

BOOKINGS & BOOKINGS MEN
Studio 6, 27A Pembridge Villas
London, W11 3EP England
T 207 221 2603 Women
T 207 229 9198 Men
F 207 229 4567
W www.bookingsmodels.co.uk
E mail@bookingsmodels.co.uk

Bruce & Brown London Kids
203 Canalot Studios, 222 Kensal Road
London, W10 5BN England
T 208 968 5585
F 208 964 0457

Childsplay • The Children's Agency
1 Cathedral Street
London, SE1 9DE England
T 207 403 4834
F 207 403 1656

Christian's Characters
London House, 266 Fulham Road, Chelsea
London, SW10 9EL England
T 207 795 3000
F 207 795 0400

CRAWFORDS
2 Conduit Street
London, W1S 2X8 England
T 207 629 6464
F 207 355 1084

Dreams International Model & Casting Agency
Empire House, 175 Picadilly, Mayfair
London, WIC 9DB England
T 207 359 4786
F 207 688 0771

F.M.
122 Brompton Road
London, SW3 1JE England
T 207 225 1355
F 207 581 2113

Gavin's Models
11 Old Burlington Street
London, W1S 3A0 England
T 207 440 5650
F 207 734 8603

GLOBAL MODEL MANAGEMENT
39-40 St James's Place
London, SW1 A1NS England
T 207 629 8407
F 207 629 8163
W www.gmmmodels.com
E gmm@gmmmodels.com

GoodFellas
122 Brompton Road
London, SW3 1JE England
T 207 584 9974
F 207 591 0238

HUGHES MODELS 12+
67A Franciscan Road, 67c
London, SW17 8DZ England
Europe's First & Foremost 12+ Agency!
T 208 672 8494
F 208 672 8494
W www.fashionfile.com
E cherylhughes1@virgin.net

IMG MODELS
Bentinck House, 3-8 Bolsover Street
London, W1P 7HG England
Contact: Jonathan Phang
T 207 580 5885
F 207 580 5868
W www.imgworld.com
***See Ad In New York Section.**

IMM LTD • INTERNATIONAL MODEL MANAGEMENT
Unit H, 21 Heathman's Road
London, SW6 4TJ England
Contact: Karsten Edwards
T 207 610 9111
F 207 736 2221
W www.internationalmodelmanagement.co.uk
E Karstenimm@aol.com

Kamera Kids
KK Studio, 9 Station Parade
London, SW12 9AZ England
T 208 675 4911
F 208 673 1364

MAVERICK MODEL MANAGEMENT LTD
134 Lots Road
London, SW10 0RJ England
T 207 823 3585
F 207 823 3586

M & P Management
3 - 4 Bentinck Street
London, WIM 5RN England
T 207 224 0560
F 207 224 0655

Model Plan
Unit 4, 3rd Flr, Harbour Yard, Chelsea Harbour
London, SW10 0X0 England
T 207 351 3244
F 207 351 2292

Models One • Models One Men
Omega House, 471-473 King's Road
London, SW10 0LU England
T 207 351 6033
F 207 376 5821

NEV'S MODELLING AGENCY
Regal House, 198 Kings Road
London, SW3 5KP England
T 207 352 9496
F 207 352 6068
W www.nevs.co.uk
E getamodel@nevs.co.uk

Next Model Management
175-179 St. Johns Street
London, EC1V4LW England
T 207 251 9850
F 207 251 9851

Ordinary People Ltd
8 Camden Road
London, NW1 9DP England
T 207 267 7007
F 207 267 5677

Premier Model Management Limited
40-42 Parker Street
London, WCB 5PQ England
T 207 333 0888
F 207 323 1221

Rage Models
256 Edgeware Road, Tigress House
London, W2 1DS England
T 207 262 0515
F 207 402 0507

Storm Model Management
5 Jubilee Place
London, SW3 3TD England
T 207 352 2278
F 207 376 5145

≫

ENGLAND

Yvonne Paul Management
10 Tiverton Road
London, NW10 3HL England
T 208 960 0022
F 208 960 0410

• • • • • • • • • •

Tuesdays Child
Gateway House, Watersgreen
Macclesfield, SK11 6LH England
T 162 561 2244
F 162 550 1765

BOSS MODEL MANAGEMENT LIMITED
Half Moon Chambers, Chapel Walks
Manchester, M2 1HN England
Contact: Debra Burns, Managing Director
T 161 834 3403
F 161 832 5219
W www.bossagencies.co.uk
E julie@bossagencies.co.uk

MMA • Manchester Model Agency
14 Albert Square
Manchester, M2 5PF England
T 161 236 1335
F 161 832 2502

Model Plan
1st Floor, Lloyds House, 18 Lloyd Street
Manchester, M2 5WA England
T 161 819 1083
F 161 819 1180

Babies, Tots, Teens & 20's
Hampton House, 33 Church Drive
N Harrow, Middlesex, HA2 7NR England
T 208 429 3030

MODEL & TALENT AGENCIES

ESTONIA • COUNTRY CODE: 372

BEATRICE MASS MODEL MANAGEMENT
Roosikrantsi 4C
Tallinn, 10119 Estonia
Contact: Raul Andresson
T 6 466 226
T 5 145 600 GSM
F 6 314 177
W www.mass.ee
E mass@mass.ee

GAITHEL STYLE
Aedvilja 4
Tallinn, 10919 Estonia
Contact: Artur Hallik, Manager
T 5394 2297
E gaithel@hotmail.com

HARTMAN MODEL MANAGEMENT
AiA 21-17
Tallinn, 10111 Estonia
T 641 8625
F 641 8624
W www.hartman.ee
E sigrid.hartman@mail.ee

Modelnet
Parnu Mnt. 21
Tallin, EE001 Estonia
T 6 266 430
F 6 266 431

MODEL & TALENT AGENCIES

FINLAND • COUNTRY CODE: 358

Helsinki

OY FONDI MODELS
Unionkatu 45A
Helsinki, 00170 Finland
Contact: Eeva Ketola
T 9 684 0160
F 9 684 01626
W www.fondi.fi
E fondi@fondi.fi

PAPARAZZI MODEL MANAGEMENT
Salomomkatu 17 B 30
Helsinki, 00100 Finland
Contact: Laila Snellman, Managing Director
T 9 686 6410
F 9 686 64120
W www.paparazzi.fi
E mail@paparazzi.fi

PERLUCA MANAGEMENT
P.O. Box 319
Helsinki, 00151 Finland
Contact: Luca Trezzi
T 9 4541 2995
F 9 4541 2990
W www.perlucamanagement.com
E mail@perlucamanagement.com

SUOMEN EUROPE FASHION
Frederikinkatu 29 A
Helsinki, 00120 Finland
T 9 608 041
F 9 640 303
W www.sef.sci.fi
E sef@sci.fi

• • • • • • • • • •

Pariss Model Agency
Tuomikuja 7
Seinajoki, 60100 Finland
T 6 414 0137
F 6 421 2250

SUOMEN EUROPE FASHION
Satakunnankatu 14, Box 673
Tampere, 33101 Finland
T 3 2237046
F 3 2237600
W www.sef.sci.fi
E sef@sci.fi

MODEL & TALENT AGENCIES

FRANCE • COUNTRY CODE: 33

HOURRA! MODELS
333 Corniche Kennedy
Marseille, 13007 France
Contact: Michele Lori
T 4 9 77 70 70
F 4 96 11 04 11
W www.hourra-models.com
E HOURRA-MARSEILLE@wanadoo.fr

Fam International
30 Bd Vital Bouhot
Neuilly, 92521 France
T 1 41 92 06 50
F 1 46 37 45 50

HOURRA! MODELS
28 rue de la Buffa
Nice, 06000 France
Contact: Eric Lafont
T 4 93 88 00 99
F 4 93 82 51 51
W www.hourra-models.com
E HOURRA@wanadoo.fr

Paris

Absolu
50 rue Etienne Marcel,
Paris, 75002 France
T 1 44 76 58 90
F 1 44 76 58 91

Bananas Mambo
9 rue Duphot
Paris, 75001 France
T 1 40 20 02 03
F 1 40 20 41 20

Beauties
22 rue de Caumartin
Paris, 75009 France
T 1 47 42 51 79
F 1 47 42 01 51

BEST MEN / CIM
98 bis, Boulevard Hausmann
Paris, 75008 France
T 1 44 69 30 20
F 1 44 69 30 21

BEST WOMEN / CIM
98 bis, Boulevard Hausmann
Paris, 75008 France
T 1 44 69 30 22
F 1 44 69 30 27

City Models
21 rue Jean Mermoz
Paris, 75008 France
T 1 53 93 33 33
F 1 53 93 33 34

Click Models
27 rue Vernet
Paris, 75008 France
T 1 47 23 44 00
F 1 47 20 31 15

CONTREBANDE
48 rue Sainte-Anne
Paris, 75002 France
Contact: Eric Perceval
Model Agency - Lic. Number 98
Artistic Agent - Lic. Number 884
T 1 40 20 42 20
F 1 40 20 42 21
W www.contrebande.com
E booking@contrebande.com
***See Ad This Section.**

Crystal Model Agency
9 rue Duphot
Paris, 75001 France
T 1 42 61 98 98
F 1 42 61 90 47

ELITE MODEL MANAGEMENT
8 bis rue Lecuirot
Paris, 75014 France
T 1 40 44 32 22
F 1 40 44 32 80

≥≥

FORD MODELS
9 rue Scribe
Paris, 75009 France
T 1 53 05 25 25
F 1 53 05 25 26
W www.fordmodelseurope.com

IDOLE MODEL MANAGEMENT
3, rue du Cirque
Paris, 75008 France
Contact: Michel Jouneau
T 1 53 96 06 00
F 1 53 96 06 01
W www.idole.com
E agence@idole.com

IMG MODELS
16, avenue de l'Opera
Paris, 75001 France
Contact: Jeni Rose
T 1 55 35 12 00
F 1 55 35 12 01
W www.imgworld.com
E tbonneav@imgworld.com
***See Ad In New York Section.**

Karin Models
9 Avenue Hoche
Paris, 75008 France
T 1 45 63 08 23
F 1 45 63 58 18

Madison Models
4 Avenue Hoche
Paris, 75008 France
T 1 44 29 26 36
F 1 47 63 44 04

Marilyn Agency
4 rue de la Paix
Paris, 75002 France
T 1 53 29 53 53
F 1 53 29 53 00

MGM
4 rue de la Paix
Paris, 75002 France
T 1 53 29 53 39
F 1 53 29 53 02

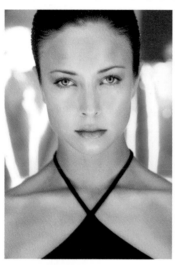

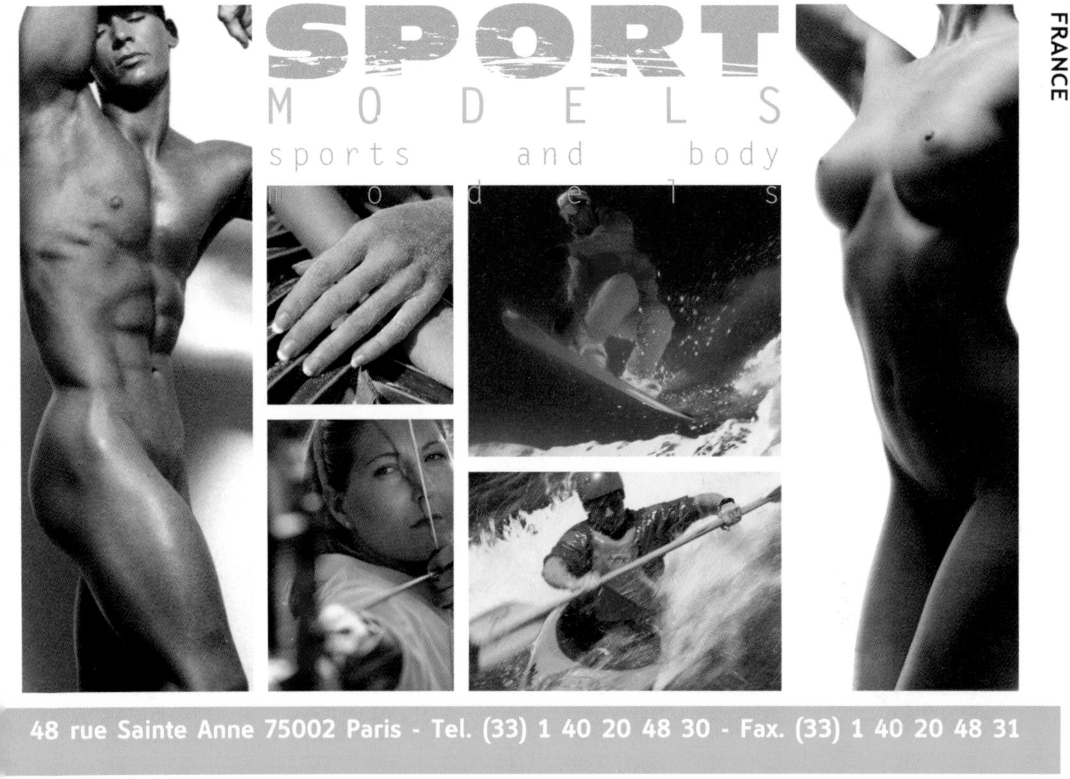
SPORT
MODELS
sports and body models
48 rue Sainte Anne 75002 Paris - Tel. (33) 1 40 20 48 30 - Fax. (33) 1 40 20 48 31

Men of Karin
9 Avenue Hoche
Paris, 75008 France
T 1 45 63 33 69
F 1 45 63 17 71

Metropolitan Models
7 Bd des Capucines
Paris, 75002 France
T 1 42 66 52 85
F 1 42 66 48 75

NATHALIE MODEL AGENCY
10 Rue Daubigny
Paris, 75017 France
Contact: Nathalie Cros Coitton, Director
T 1 44 29 07 10
F 1 44 29 07 11
W www.nathalie-models.com
E nathalie@nathalie-models.com

NEXT MANAGEMENT
188, rue de Rivoli
Paris, 75001 France
T 1 53 45 13 00
F 1 53 45 13 01
W www.nextmodels.com

People Agency
11 Rue Richepanse
Paris, 75008 France
T 1 55 35 09 90
F 1 55 35 09 95

PH ONE INTERNATIONAL MODEL AGENCY
50 rue Etienne Marcel
Paris, 75002 France
T 1 44 76 58 70
F 1 44 74 58 71

Profil
11 rue des Arquebusiers
Paris, 75003 France
T 1 40 29 04 04
F 1 42 78 23 88

REBECCA
33 rue du Petit Musc
Paris, 75004 France
T 1 44 61 84 20
F 1 44 61 84 21

SILVESTRE MODEL MANAGEMENT
70 Boulevard Sebastopol
Paris, 75003 France
T 1 44 54 18 18
F 1 44 54 18 19

>>

Slides
9 rue Duphot
Paris, 75001 France
T 1 42 61 18 08
F 1 42 61 90 47

SPORT MODELS
48 rue Sainte-Anne
Paris, 75002 France
Contact: Eric Perceval
T 1 40 20 48 30
F 1 40 20 48 31
W www.sport-models.com
E desk@sport-models.com
***See Ad This Section.**

Success Steff
64 rue Rambuteau
Paris, 75003 France
T 1 44 54 94 00
F 1 42 78 17 67

Vision Agency
11 rue des Arquebusiers
Paris, 75003 France
T 1 4454 9400
F 1 4278 1767

• • • • • • • • • •

ZENITH MODELS
B.P. 35
Strasbourg Cedex 2, 67031 France
Contact: Jean-Frederic Schaller
T 388 56 20 40
F 388 56 38 39
W www.zenithmodels.com
E info@zenithmodels.com

MODEL & TALENT AGENCIES

GERMANY • COUNTRY CODE: 49

Berlin

Bandits Model Management
Widosteig 15
Berlin, 12524 Germany
T 171 311 93 21
F 30 6397 5550

FAMOUS INTERNATIONAL MODEL AGENCY
Spreeufer 5
Berlin, 10178 Germany
Contact: Helmuth Lang
T 30 327 5556
F 30 324 8064
W www.famousagency.com
E models@famousagency.com

Kunstlerdienst Berlin
Kurfuerstendamm 210
Berlin, 10719 Germany
T 30 88 43050
F 30 88 430562

M4 Management
Torstraffe 125
Berlin, 10119 Germany
T 30 275 6210
F 30 279 6463

TYPE FACE
Tempelhofer Ufer 10
Berlin, 10963 Germany
Contact: Inka / Bettina
T 30 283 9850
F 30 2839 8529
W www.type-face.de
E info@type-face.de

Viva Models
Hackefcher Markt 3
Berlin, 10178 Germany
T 30 881 9111
F 30 240 8989

Dusseldorf

Bond Models Model Management Gmbh
Fuerstenwall 182
Dusseldorf, 40215 Germany
T 211 3850007
F 211 3858700

Cockroach
Ahnfeldstr 45
Düsseldorf, 40239 Germany
T 211 639 9096
F 211 639 9098

D'SELECTION
Cecilien Allee 66
Düsseldorf, 40474 Germany
T 211 84555
F 211 84550
W www.d-selection.com
E office@d-selection.com

E Models Management
Corneliusstr 71
Düsseldorf, 40215 Germany
T 211 386 100
F 211 386 1010

MODEL POOL
Akademiestr 7
Düsseldorf, 40123 Germany
T 211 865 560
F 211 865 5665
W www.model-pool.de
E info@model-pool.de

NO TOYS
Schwanenmarkt 12
Düsseldorf, 40213 Germany
T 211 322 100
F 211 322 111
W www.notoys.de
E sylvia@notoys.de

STARS MODEL MANAGEMENT GMBH
Benrather Strasse 6
Düsseldorf, 40213 Germany
Contact: Maggie Gaul & Angelika Hess
T 211 86 56 10
F 211 32 34 34

Frankfurt

East West Models
Launitzstr 12
Frankfurt, 60594 Germany
T 69 6109 310
F 69 6109 3131

Frankfurt One!
Hamburger Alee 45
Frankfurt, 60486 Germany
T 69 975 8750
F 69 975 875 75

Kunstlerdienst
Saonestr 2-4
Frankfurt/M, 60528 Germany
T 69 6670 0
F 69 6670 459

S'MS • SEEBER
Darmstädter Landstr 320
Frankfurt, 60598 Germany
T 69 685 005
F 011 49 69 689 7282
W www.sms.modelagency.de
E sms@modell.de

>>

Hamburg

AQUARIUS MODELS
Schauenburger Strasse 15
Hamburg, D-20095 Germany
Contact: Gert Mueller
T 40 32 81 08 82
F 40 32 81 08 81
E aquariusmo@aol.com

BODY & SOUL
WerderstraBe 39
Hamburg, 20144 Germany
Contact: Pia Kohles
T 40 41 2091
F 40 410 4748
E info@bodyandsoulmodels.de

HOEPPEL AGENCY
Lokstedler Steindamm 31
Hamburg, 22529 Germany
We represent local talent in Hamburg from Kids to Young Adults.
T 40 566 061
F 40 560 1810

Kunstlerdienst Hamburg
Nagelsweg 9
Hamburg, 20097 Germany
T 40 24 850
F 40 24 851 457

LOUISA MODELS HAMBURG
Feldbrunnen Strasse 24
Hamburg, 20148 Germany
Contact: Louisa Von Minckwitz, Agent
T 40 414 40 100 Booking
T 40 414 40 111 Make-Up
F 40 414 40 222
W www.louisa-models.de
E info-ham@louisa-models.de

M4 Models
Schluterstr 54a
Hamburg, 20146 Germany
T 40 413 2360
F 40 413 23616

Mega Model Agency
Kaiser-Wilhelm-Str 93
Hamburg, 20355 Germany
T 40 355 2200
F 40 355 2202 2

Model Contact
Borsteler Bogen 27
Hamburg, 22453 Germany
T 40 553 8885
F 40 553 8886

Model Management Hamburg
Hartungstr 5
Hamburg, 20146 Germany
T 40 440 555
F 40 450 0885

MODEL TEAM
Schluterstrasse 60
Hamburg, 20146 Germany
Contact: Soni Ekvall
T 40 414 1037
F 40 414 1033 4
E modelteamhh@hotmail.com

MODELWERK
Rothenbaumchaussee 3
Hamburg, 20148 Germany
T 40 44 79 29
F 40 44 79 10
W www.modelwerk.com
E modelwerk@modelwerk.com

NETWORK MODELS
Milchstrasse 26
Hamburg, 20148 Germany
T 40 44 1451
F 40 45 7114
W www.network-models.de
E info@network-models.de

OKAY MODELS
Ost West Strasse 63
Hamburg, 20457 Germany
Contact: Maggie Fedorow-Berndt
T 40 378 5000
F 40 378 5001 0
W www.okaymodels.de
E okaymodels@aol.com

PEOPLE & FRIENDS
Gerhofstr 29
Hamburg, 20354 Germany
T 40 357 6440
F 40 357 64444
W www.peopleandfriends.de
E anneca@peopleandfriends.de

Promod Model Agency
Barmbeker Str 136
Hamburg, 22299 Germany
T 40 471 0000
F 40 471 0002 2

TALENTS MODEL AGENCY
Isestr. 43
Hamburg, 20144 Germany
Contact: Daniel Schmitt-Eisleben

WOLF MODELS
Alsterufer 46
Hamburg, D-20354 Germany
Contact: Wolf Lueck
T 40 413 3190
F 40 413 31941
W www.wolfmodels.de
E wolfmodels@t-online.de

XS Excess Model Management Gmbh
Heimhuderstr 18
Hamburg, 20148 Germany
T 40 450 377 10
F 40 450 377 15

• • • • • • • • • •

Model Point
Koenigstor 43
Kassel, 34117 Germany
T 561 772220
F 561 772224

Supreme Model Agency
Waldparkstrobe 30
Mannheim, 68163 Germany
T 621 833 2330
F 621 833 2339

München

AGENTUR BRIGITTE
Leopoldstrasse 27
München, 80821 Germany
T 89 745 02 840
F 89 745 02 841

Cawi Models
Schwanthalerstrasse 13
München , 80336 Germany
T 89 557 995
F 89 550 122

Harry's Model Management
Virchowstrasse 2
München, 80805 Germany
T 89 360 0000
F 89 361 7067

Kunstlerdienst München
Sonnenstr 2/IV
München, 80331 Germany
T 89 54 45 1130
F 89 54 45 1154

LOUISA MODELS MUNCHEN
Ebersberger Strasse 9
München, 81679 Germany
Contact: Louisa Von Minckwitz. Agent
T 89 9210 9620 Women
T 89 9210 9630 Men
T 89 9210 9641 Make-Up
F 89 9210 9638
W www.louisa-models.de
E info-muc@louisa-models.de

MUNICH MODELS
Siegfriedstrasse 17
München, 80803 Germany
T 89 3899 830
F 89 3899 8333
W www.munich-models.de
E booking@munich-models.de

NOVA MODELS
Antonienstr 3
München, 80802 Germany
Contact: Auja Reiling, Headbooker
T 89 3839 1819 Men + Women
F 89 38 39 1888
W www.nova-models.de
E girl@nova-models.de
E men@nova-models.de

PS Model Management Munich
Holzstrasse 12
München, 80469 Germany
T 89 291 9230
F 89 291 92350

Smile Model Management
Konradinstrasse 10
München , 81543 Germany
T 89 624 0000
F 89 624 00044

TALENTS MUNCHEN
Ohmstr 5
München, 80802 Germany
T 89 3883 7730
F 89 3883 7733
W www.talents-models.com
E sylvia@talents-models.com

UNITY MODELS
Friedrichstrasse 31
München , 80801 Germany
T 89 344 740
F 89 3300 8711
W www.unity-models.com
E team@unity-models.com

• • • • • • • • • •

>>

TODAYS MODELS
Moltkestr 15
Nürnberg, 90429 Germany
T 911 28 8948
F 911 28 8988

Stuttgart

First Agency
Sophienstr 19
Stuttgart, 70178 Germany
T 711 60 0030
F 711 60 0090

Kunstlerdienst Stuttgart
Jägerstr 14-16
Stuttgart, 70174 Germany
T 711 941 0
F 711 941 2401

RITA JAEGER MODELS
Rotebuehltlat 29
Stuttgart, 70178 Germany
T 711 226 2051
F 711 226 3895

Rothchild
Böblinger Str 10b
Stuttgart, 70178 Germany
T 711 603 040
F 711 640 0802

• • • • • • • • • •

Le Visage
Petrusstr 19a
Trier, 54214 Germany
T 651 2 5463
F 651 2 5463

GLOBAL PROFESSIONAL GROUP
Sooderstrasse 23
Wiesbaden, D-65193 Germany
Contact: Oliver Darenberg
T 611 9 54 41 44 Women
T 611 9 54 41 45 Men
F 611 9 54 40 32
W www.gpg-darenberg.de
E info@gpg-darenberg.de

GREECE • COUNTRY CODE: 30

Athens

ACE MODEL MANAGEMENT
9, Irodotou Str
Athens, 10674 Greece
Contact: Mara Matridimopoulou, Managing Director
T 1 725 8531
T 1 725 8532
T 1 725 8533
F 1 721 8963
E ace1@ath.forthnet.gr

ACTION MANAGEMENT
Ferekidou 14-16
Athens, 116 36 Greece
Contact: Dotte Klingström, Director
or Anthi Lalou, Manager
T 1 751 8080
F 1 751 2047
W www.action-management.com
E actionmg@otenet.gr

AGENCE IMAGE MANAGEMENT
44 Ipsilandoy Str
Athens, Kolonaki 10676 Greece
Contact: Antigone Deliou
T 1 729 2611
F 1 721 3354
W www.agence.gr
E agence@agence.gr

Alice Models and Fashion Show Organization
70, Kiprou Street
Athens, 16674 Greece
T 1 968 1730
F 1 968 1730

ELENA MODEL MANAGEMENT
22, Vasileos Georgiou B22
Athens, 11635 Greece
T 1 722 3384
F 1 724 5382

Fashion Cult
Iperidou 5
Athens, 105 58 Greece
T 1 322 1301
F 1 322 8281

Models One
4 Koumbari Street
Athens, 10674 Greece
T 1 364 5011
F 1 364 3077

M'SH • MODEL MANAGEMENT
19 Filellinon Street, 4th Floor
Athens, 10557 Greece
Contact: Yiannis Stamopoulos, Managing Director
T 1 322 4745
F 1 322 4855
E mshhouse@netor.gr

PRESTIGE GROUP MANAGEMENT S.A.
154 Syngrou Avenue
Athens, 17671 Greece
Contact: Nikos Voglis, Owner
T 1 924 4552
F 1 921 5596
E prestige@ath.forthnet.gr

Twins Models Agency
11, 25 Martiou Str, Halandri
Athens, 152 32 Greece
T 1 685 6200
F 1 685 6201

• • • • • • • • • •

UNIVERSAL ARTISTS / MODELS
27 Aetorahis
Thessaloniki, 54640 Greece
Contact: Mike Harris
T 31 82 1742
F 31 81 9424
E interalex@hol.gr

MODEL & TALENT AGENCIES

GUAM • COUNTRY CODE: 67

John Robert Powers
P.O. Box 96, Ada Prof'l Comm'l Center, Suite 201
Agana, 96932 Guam
T 477 9647
F 477 7029

MODEL & TALENT AGENCIES

HONG KONG • COUNTRY CODE: 852

Cal Carrie's
Anton Commercial Centre
2-12 Queen's Road West, Sheung Wan
Hong Kong, Hong Kong
T 2543 3380
F 2543 3830

Catwalk Productions Ltd
Cornell Centre, 50 Wing Tai Road Room 1702, Chai Wan,
Hong Kong, Hong Kong
T 2598 0663
F 2598 9719

ELITE HK MODEL MANAGEMENT HOLDINGS LTD
Suite 901, Workington Tower
78 Bonham Strand East
Sheung Wan, Hong Kong
Contact: Paul Lau, General Manager
T 2850 5550
F 2851 3384
E elitehk@vol.net

Kitty's Modelling & Production Consultant
1-3 Burrows Street,
Bel Trade Commercial Bldg, 4/F, Wan Chai
Hong Kong, Hong Kong
T 572 9788
F 572 7544

MODELS INTERNATIONAL LTD
26/F, 128 Lockhart Road, Wanchai
Hong Kong, Hong Kong
Contact: Candy Chan
T 2529 6183
F 2865 2381
W www.modelshk.com
E booking@modelshk.com

NEW FACE MODEL AGENCY • HONG KONG
1F, No 62, Wellington St, Central
Hong Kong, Hong Kong
Contact: Paul Chang
T 2536 9911
F 2526 6788
W www.newface-model.com.tw
E newface@netvigator.com
***See Ad This Section.**

Signal 8 Model Management
68-70 Wellington Street,
9B Kai Wah Building, Central
Hong Kong, Hong Kong
T 2523 1025
F 2884 9082

STARZ PEOPLE (HK) LTD
Unit 503-504, 5/F, 1 Lyndhurst Tower
I Lyndhurst Terrace, Central,
Hong Kong, Hong Kong
Contact: Mee-Yian Yong
T 2536 0225
F 2536 0333
W www.starz.com.hk
E starzhk@netvigator.com

Irene's Model Booking Svc Ltd
105-111 Thomson Road,
Harvard Comm Building Flat B, 14F
Wanchai, Hong Kong
T 2891 7667
F 2838 4840

MODEL & TALENT AGENCIES

HUNGARY • COUNTRY CODE: 36

Budapest

ATTRACTIVE ELITE MODELS
Kadar Utca 9-11
Budapest, H-1132 Hungary
Contact: Orsi Feher / Marta Haklik
T 1 236 4022
T 30 200 7291
F 1 236 4023
W www.modelbase.net/attractive
E attractive@modelbase.net

FASHION MODELS
Andrassy Ut 36, 1st Floor
Budapest, 1061 Hungary
Contact: Alex Pocsai / Andrew Ali
T 1 354 0029
F 1 354 0029
W www.fashionmodels.hu
E office@fashionmodels.hu

IMAGE MODEL MANAGEMENT
Bródy Sándor u.9
Budapest, 1088 Hungary
T 1 338 1099
F 1 318 7321
W www.image.hu
E image@image.hu

L & W Model Agency
Sopron ut 40
Budapest, 1117 Hungary
T 1 203 9159
F 1 203 5897

MODEL & TALENT AGENCIES

ICELAND • COUNTRY CODE: 36

Eskimo Models
Ingolfsstraeti 1A
Reykjavik, 101 Iceland
T 552 8012
F 552 8011

GENAGE MODEL MANAGEMENT
Holmgardur 34
Reykjavik, 108 Iceland
Contact: Mr. Ingi Karlsson
T 553 4070
F 553 4072
W www.genagemodels.com
E office@genagemodels.com

Icelandic Models
Skeifan 7
Reykjavik, 108 Iceland
T 588 7727
F 588 7797

MODEL & TALENT AGENCIES

INDONESIA • COUNTRY CODE: 62

John Robert Powers
Komplek Sudirman Agung Blok B-08,
Jl Panglimna Besar Sudirman
Bali, Denpasar, 80225 Indonesia
T 361 242 933

Elite Indonesia
Graha Darya Varia 3rd B Floor
93, Jalan Melawai Raya
Jakarta, 12130 Indonesia
T 217 261 040
F 217 261 031

John Robert Powers
Central Cikini Bldg, JL Cikini Raya No. 60V
Jakarta, 10330 Indonesia
T 21 314 0541
F 21 310 0353

John Robert Powers
Jl. Brigjend. Katamso 717 B
Medan, Indonesia
T 1 769 788
F 1 553 693

John Robert Powers
Jl. Slamet Riyadi 33
Solo, 57112 Indonesia
T 271 664 516
F 271 664 518

MODEL & TALENT AGENCIES

IRELAND • COUNTRY CODE: 353

Dublin

AMBERS MODEL AGENCY
184 Rathfarnham Road
Dublin, 14 Ireland
T 353 1 490 1405
F 353 1 490 6529

First Option Model Management
40 Dame Street
Dublin , 2 Ireland
T 1 670 5233
F 1 670 5261

Geraldine Brand Agency
Ashdown House, 565 Howth Road, Raheny
Dublin, 5 Ireland
T 1 832 7332

Impact Models
P.O. Box 7534, Cardiff Lane
Dublin, 2 Ireland
T 1 295 4095

MORGAN, THE AGENCY
13 Herbert Place
Dublin, 2 Ireland
T 353 1 661 4572
F 353 1 662 4575

Network 2000 Modelling Agency
721 S Circular Road
Dublin, 8 Ireland
T 1 671 7055

• • • • • • • • • •

Access Model Agency
17 Sandycove Point
Sandycove, Ireland
T 1 280 7450

MODEL & TALENT AGENCIES

ISRAEL • COUNTRY CODE: 972

Sarit Damir
79 Bialik St
Ramat-Gan, 52511 Israel
T 3 751 7946
F 3 575 2568

Tel Aviv

IMAGE MODELS AGENCY
118 Ehad Haam Street
Tel Aviv, 65208 Israel
Contact: Betty Rockway
T 3 685 0999
F 3 685 1011
W www.image-models.com
E image1@netvision.net.il

KARIN MODELS
3 Nafcha St, Shenkin Corner
Tel Aviv, Israel
Contact: Ofer Raphaeli
T 3 620 8808
F 3 620 8807
W www.karinmodels.co.il
E info@karinmodels.co.il

Look Models & Talent
35 Bnei Brak Street, 4th Floor
Tel Aviv, 66021 Israel
T 3 638 6900
F 3 638 6940

YULI MODELS
1 Yordey Hasira St
Tel Aviv, 63508 Israel
T 3 544 6151
F 3 544 6152
W www.yulimodels.com
E info@yulimodels.com

MODEL & TALENT AGENCIES

ITALY • COUNTRY CODE: 39

COLLECTION MODEL MANAGEMENT
Via Pancaldi 5
Bologna, 40138 Italy
Contact: Stefano Cavezzi, Managing Director
T 051 343 442
T 051 346 688
F 051 391 681
W www.collectionmodels.com
E info@collectionmodels.com

Milano

Christian Jacques Women • CJ Men
Via Tortona 14,
Milano, 20144 Italy
T 02 5810 7440
F 02 5811 3677

ELITE MODEL MANAGEMENT SRL
Via S. Vittore 40
Milano, 20123 Italy
T 02 467 521
F 02 481 9058
W www.elite.it
E elite@elite.it

EYE FOR I MODEL MANAGEMENT
Via Guerrazzi, 1
Milano, 20145 Italy
Contact: Patti Piazzi
T 02 345 471 Print
F 02 3454 7222 Print Fax
T 02 3453 5144 Runway
F 02 3453 4128 Runway Fax
T 02 3454 7210 Accounting
F 02 3454 7222
W www.eyefori.com
E patti@eyefori.com

≫

ITALY

Flash Models Management
Via Tortona 14
Milano, 20144 Italy
T 02 837 3010
F 02 837 2221

Funny Type
Via Aurello Saffi No 11
Milano, 20123 Italy
T 02 461 487
F 02 498 4525

FUTURE MODEL MEN
Via Voghera 25
Milano, 20144 Italy
Contact: Wal Torres
T 02 833 0101
F 02 8330 1029
W www.futuremodelmen.com
E info@futuremodelmen.com

ICE MODEL MANAGEMENT
Via G G Mora 2
Milano, 20123 Italy
T 02 833 880
F 02 8942 9171

JOY MODEL MANAGEMENT
Via San Vittore 40
Milano, 20123 Italy
Contact: Maristella Becucci
T 02 4800 2776
F 02 4802 2598
W www.joymodels.com
E joy@joymodels.com

Look Now
Via A. Da Giussano, 16
Milano, 20145 Italy
T 02 4802 0126
F 02 498 1586

PAOLO TOMEI MODELS
Via Voghera 25
Milano, 20144 Italy
Contact: Paolo Tomei
T 02 833 0101
F 02 8330 1030
W www.paolotomeimodels.com
E info@paolotomeimodels.com

PEPEA MODEL MANAGEMENT
Via Solari 11
Milano, 20144 Italy
Contact: Giorgio Riviera, Head Booker
T 02 8942 0135
F 02 8942 9371
E pepeamodel@hotmail.com

WANT MODEL MANAGEMENT
Via Borgonuovo, 10, 2nd Floor
Milano, 20121 Italy
Contact: Paola Redaelli
T 02 290 6631
F 02 2901 4477
W www.wantmodel.it
E info@wantmodelmanagement.com

Why Not
Via Zenale 9
Milano, 20123 Italy
T 02 485 331
F 02 481 8342

ZOOM MODEL MANAGEMENT
Via Franchetti 2
Milano, 20124 Italy
Contact: Andrea Tradico
T 02 657 0669
T 02 657 0749
F 02 657 0760
E zoommodel@tiscalinet.it

GAP Model Management
Via Valadier, 36
Roma, 00193 Italy
T 06 322 0108
F 06 321 9371

MODEL & TALENT AGENCIES

JAPAN • COUNTRY CODE: 81

Central Fashion Co Ltd
3F Cinq Ishikawabashi Bldg,
5-18 Dankei-dori, Mizuho-ku
Nagoya, 467 Japan
T 52 836 6663
F 52 836 6667

Osaka

COSMOPOLITAN MODEL AGENCY CO. LTD.
Asahi Plaza Umeda 714
4-11 Tsuruno-cho, Kita-Ku
Osaka, 530-0014 Japan
Contact: Keiko Hatano
T 6 6359 5067
F 6 6377 3040
W www.cosmopolitanagency.com
E cosmopolitan@mua.biglobe.ne.jp

FORZA INC
Torishima Office One Building
1-5-2 Temma, Kita-Ku
Osaka, 530-0043 Japan
Contact: Mika Hirayama
T 6 6882 7200
F 6 6882 7205
W www.forzamodels.co.jp
E agency@forzamodels.co.jp
***See Ad This Section.**

John Robert Powers
9F Urban Life Bldg, 4-3-4 Chome Midousuji,
Minamisenba, Chuo-Ku
Osaka, 542-0081 Japan
T 6 241 0773

Select Men Model Management
1-2-2-200 Umeda, Kita-ku
Osaka, 530-0001 Japan
T 6 6344 6346
F 6 6344 6295

VISAGE • JAPAN
1-2-2-200 Umada, Kita-Ku
Osaka, 530 Japan
Contact: Keiko Hara
T 6 6348 1855
F 6 6348 1858
W www5b.biglobe.ne.jp/~visage/
E visage@muj.biglobe.ne.jp

ZEM INC
Osaka Ekimae No. 2 Bldg. 2F
1-2-2-200 Umeda, Kita-ku
Osaka 530-0001 Japan
Contact: Tami Chiba, Managing Director
T 6 6341 5252
F 6 6341 1907
E zemz@mvj.biglobe.ne.jp

Tokyo

Amazone
403 Harajuku Coop,
1-14-14 Jingumea, Shibuya-ku
Toyko, Japan
T 3 3423 0644
F 3 3423 6753

AGENCE PRESSE MODEL MANAGEMENT
6F Maison Blanche, 5-6-6 Aoyama Heights
Minami-Aoyama, Minato-ku
Tokyo, 107 Japan
Contact: Rika Hashimoto
T 3 3406 6771
F 3 3406 5081
E agence@mue.biglobe.ne.jp

ARTS C MODELS
305 Tvses Part 6
1-9-18 Minami Ikebukuro, Toshima-ku
Toyko, 171-0022 Japan
Contact: Atsushi Miyakoshi
T 3 5396 8819
F 3 5396 8819
W www.artscmodels.com
E artsc@pa3.so-net.ne.jp

AVENUE 1 CO. LTD
5F M-Bldg, 7-9-7 Akasaka, Minato-ku
Tokyo, Japan
Contact: Sawa Saito, Director
T 3 5570 1168
F 3 5570 1154
E avenue@on.rim.or.jp
***See Ad This Section.**

>>

AXELLE INC
Root Higashiazabu 10F
3-4-18, Higashiazabu, Minato-Ku
Tokyo, 106-0044 Japan
Contact: Keiko Kyomoto, President
T 3 3582 1212
F 3 3582 6430
W www.axelle.co.jp
E model@axelle.co.jp

Bon' Image
7-3-16 #303 Roppongi, Minato-ku
Tokyo, Japan
T 3 3403 4110
F 3 3403 4662

BRAVO models

BRAVO MODELS
Room 701, 3-1-25 NishiAzabu, Minatoku
Tokyo, 106-0031 Japan
Contact: Shoko Arai, President
T 3 3746 9090
F 3 3746 9901
W www.bravomodels.net
E shoko@bravomodels.net

CINQ DEUX UN CO., LTD.
Al Bergo Nogizaka 508
9-6-28 Akasaka, Minato-ku
Tokyo, 107-0052 Japan
Contact: Machiko Arikura
T 3 3402 8445 Women
T 3 3402 7591 Men
T 3 3402 8688 Prima
F 3 3402 8687
E cdujapan@blue.ocn.ne.jp
*See Ad This Section.

DONNA INC
503, 1-7-9 Jinnan, Shibuya-Ku
Tokyo 150-0041 Japan
Contact: Junko Shimazaki
T 3 3770 8255
F 3 3770 8266
E donna@nn.iij4u.or.jp

EVVIVA INC
Akasaka Tokyu Bldg 5-F
2-14-3 Nagatacho, Chiyoda-ku
Tokyo, 100-0014 Japan
Contact: Ríe Aizawa
T 3 3502 4721
F 3 3502 4720
E evviva@mint.ocn.ne.jp

Faces Guild Modeling Agency
1-8-13 Nishi-Azabu, Minato-ku
Tokyo, Japan
T 3 3475 0152
F 3 3475 5687

FOLIO
1-10-10, 5F, Azabujuban, Minato-Ku
Tokyo, 106-0045 Japan
Contact: Yumi Sakai
T 3 3586 6481
F 3 3505 2980
E folio@mb.kcom.ne.jp

FORZA INC
Nogizaka Park Front Building 5F
1-15-15 Minami-Aoyama, Minato-ku
Tokyo, 107-0062 Japan
Contact: Mika Hirayama
T 3 3478 2760
F 3 3478 2761
W www.forzamodels.co.jp
E tokyo@forzamodels.co.jp
*See Ad This Section.

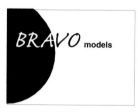

FRIDAY MODEL AGENCY
901 Star Plaza Aoyama, 1-10-3 Shibuya, Shibuya-ku
Tokyo, 150-0002 Japan
Contact: Junko (Jap Dev) / Nikki (Intl Dev)
T 3 3406 1487 International Development
T 3 3406 1550 Japanese Development
F 3 3406 1456
W www.fridaymodels.net
E info@fridaymodels.net

GALLERY MODELS
Fine Aoyama Building 8F
6-2-13 Minami Aoyama, Minato-ku
Tokyo, 107-0062 Japan
Contact: Tomoko Takeshi or Samuel Heriche
T 3 3486 4755
F 3 3486 4757
W www.gallerymodels.co.jp
E gallery@mb2.cyberoz.net

John Robert Powers
4-1 Kioi-Cho, New Otani Hotel, Chiyoda-ku
Tokyo, Japan
T 3 3221 2980
F 3 3221 2685

KIRARA JAPAN MODEL MANAGEMENT
402 St Rope Minami Aoyama
6-3-14 Minami Aoyama, Minato-ku
Tokyo, 107-0062 Japan
Contact: Suzuyo Fukuda
T 3 5466 8802
F 3 5466 8821
E kirara@mail.webnik.ne.jp

Pueblo Models
55-7-303 Motoyoyogi, Suite 303, Shibuya-ku
Tokyo, 151-0062 Japan
T 3 3468 1051
F 3 3468 1038

Satoru Model Management
Belaire Gardens 5A, 4-2-11 Jingumae, Shibuya-ku
Tokyo, 150 Japan
T 3 3475 0555
F 3 3408 7211

Tateoka Office
6-34-14 Jingumae, Room 403, Shibuya-ku,
Tokyo, 150 Japan
T 3 5466 2902
F 3 5466 2904

TEAM INC
Akasaka Tokyu Bldg 5F
2-14-3 Nagatacho, Chiyoda-ku
Tokyo, 100-0014 Japan
Contact: Kimiko Tamagawa (Men)
or Yu Ogino (Women)
T 3 3502 4711
F 3 3502 4715
E team@coral.ocn.ne.jp

Urban Agency Co Ltd
Pare Nogizaka 603, 9-5-26 Akasaka, Minato-ku
Tokyo, 107 Japan
T 3 3475 0453
F 3 3475 0529

Voice Model Management
Ph Tanaka Tamuracho Bldg,
2-12-15 Shimbashi, Minato-ku
Toyko, 105-0004 Japan
T 3 5251 5688
F 3 5251 5689

>>

JAPAN

WORLD TOP INC
2-1-4 Ebisuminami
PS Heights, Suite 3F, Shibuya-ku
Toyko, 150 Japan
Contact: Hiromi Tashiro
T 3 3719 7751
F 3 3719 8980
W www.worldtopmodels.net
E worldone@serenade.plala.or.jp
E worldtop15@hotmail.com

Y.O. Models
5-4-24 Minami Aoyama, Suite 302, Minato-ku
Tokyo, 107-0062 Japan
T 3 5467 0260
F 3 5467 0263

YOSHIE INC
#403 Gold Bldg
1-12-23 Taishido, Setagaya-ku
Tokyo, 154-0004 Japan
Contact: Yoshie Furuya
T 3 5481 2224
F 3 5481 5832
E yf01-yos@kt.rim.or.jp

ZUCCA MODEL AGENCY
Raffiné Tomigaya 601
2-20-1 Tomigaya, Shibuya-ku
Tokyo, 151-0063 Japan
Contact: Kumiko Ueno
T 3 3465 5851
F 3 3465 4871
E zucca@trio.plala.or.jp

MODEL & TALENT AGENCIES

KOREA • COUNTRY CODE: 82

Seoul

AL INTERNATIONAL MODEL AGENCY
#133-15 Kum-Hark B/D, 6F, Suite 601
Nonhyun Dong, Kangnam-gu
Seoul, Korea
T 2 597 8576
F 2 597 8573
E manageal@hotmail.com

C.A.T. THE CULTURE PRODUCTION CO LTD
#3-20, 3F, Iirae B/D
Chung Dam-Dong, Kang Nam-ku
Seoul, 135-010 Korea
Contact: Haeng Rok Jung, President
T 2 518 6437
F 2 512 5199
E catwalk@thrunet.com

Channel M Entertainemnt
13-18 So-mang B/D, 2nd Floor,
Nonhyun-dong, Kangnam-Gu,
Seoul, Korea
T 2 3442 4582
F 2 3442 4584

hershe entertainment
www.hershee.com

HERSHE MODELS
4th Floor, Shindo Bldg
48-8 Cheongdam-dong, Kangnam-gu
Seoul, 135-100 Korea
Contact: Vincent Sung / John Byun
T 2 3442 0655
F 2 3442 0656
W www.hershemodels.com
E vsung@hershee.com

Model Center International
5F Textile Center B/D,
#944-31 Daechi-3 Dong, Kangnam-Gu,
Seoul, 135-713 Korea
T 2 2528 0888
F 2 2528 0886

PRIME AGENCY CO LTD
Yuwoo B/D #402, 737-1
Hannam 2-Dong, Yongsan-Gu
Seoul, Korea
Contact: Hyun-Jin, Park or Jean Song
T 2 790 5672
F 2 790 5676
E primeagency@netsgo.com

STARS

STARS AGENCY INC
6F, Baegang Bldg, 666-14
Shinsa-Dong, Kangnam-Gu
Seoul, Korea
Contact: Jason Kim
T 2 518 1332
F 2 514 5494
W www.stars-e.com
E Jason@stars-e.com

MODEL & TALENT AGENCIES

LATVIA • COUNTRY CODE: 371

NATALIE MODEL AGENCY
27/2 Gertrudes Str
Riga, LV 1011 Latvia
Contact: Erik Meisans
T 7 312 154
F 7 312 438
W www.nataliemodels.com
E natalie@apollo.lv

MODEL & TALENT AGENCIES

MEXICO • COUNTRY CODE: 52

FACIA MODELS
Jalisco 7
Col Heroes de Padierna, CP 10700 Mexico
T 55 68 62 38
F 56 58 62 39
W www.facia.com.mx
E facia@facia.com.mx

MODELOS QUETA ROJAS
Oaxaca #96-103
Mexico City, Mexico
Contact: Enriqueta Rojas, President
T 55 11 87 55
F 55 14 28 72
W www.queta-rojas.com.mx
E queta@quetarojas.com

ARTE MODELOS
Blvd. Agua Caliente #11300 Local 225
Tijuana, BC Mexico
Contact: Enriqueta Rojas, President
T 1156 2160 06
F 1156 2162 73
W www.artemodelos.com

MODEL & TALENT AGENCIES

NICARAGUA • COUNTRY CODE: 505

SILHUETAS
Rot. Ruben Dario Km. 3 1/2 Carretera a Masaya
Managua, Nicaragua
T 278 2109
F 278 2109

MODEL & TALENT AGENCIES

NETHERLANDS • COUNTRY CODE: 31

Amsterdam

AFT Model Agency BV
Singel 117
Amsterdam, 1012 VH Netherlands
T 20 624 2628
F 20 620 6309

Company Incognito
Edisonstraat 24-1
Amsterdam, 1098 TB Netherlands
T 20 663 70 77
F 20 663 70 77

Corine's Agency
Prinsengracht 678
Amsterdam, 1017 KX Netherlands
T 20 622 67 55
F 20 620 34 09

DE BOEKERS
Herengracht 407
Amsterdam, 1017 BP Netherlands
T 20 627 27 66
F 20 622 40 78

Elite Amsterdam
Keizersgracht 448
Amsterdam, 1016 GD Netherlands
T 20 627 99 29
F 20 624 05 07

Euromodel BV
Raadhuisstraat 52
Amsterdam, 1016 DG Netherlands
T 20 623 79 57
F 20 620 36 11

THE MODEL MAKERS
Prinsengracht 343
Amsterdam, 1016 HK Netherlands
T 20 623 78 86
F 20 626 72 99

NAME MODELS
Westermarkt 2
Amsterdam, 1016 DK Netherlands
T 20 638 12 17
F 20 638 51 43

PEPERONI
Nicolaas Witsenkade 12
Amsterdam, 1017 2R Netherlands
T 20 624 4014
F 20 420 7903
W www.peperoni.net
E peperoni_net@hotmail.com

>>

NETHERLANDS

Touché Models
Herengracht 138/140
Amsterdam, 1015 BW Netherlands
T 20 625 02 54
F 20 620 48 05

Ulla Models
Weteringschans 18
Amsterdam, 1017 SG Netherlands
T 20 626 36 76
F 20 620 01 91

• • • • • • • • • •

Touche People
Bouriclusstraat 3
Arnheim, 6814 CS Netherlands
T 26 44 50 444
F 26 44 33 650

Cachet
Stratumsedijk 23G
Eindhoven, 5611 NA Netherlands
T 40 211 6900
F 40 212 7009

CREATIVE CONNECTIONS MODELS
Kleine Berg 47a
Eindhoven, 5611 EA Netherlands
Contact: Quinta De Vries, Director
T 40 2 96 03 50
F 40 2 44 54 82
W www.ccmodels.nl
E info@ccmodels.nl

Beauty People Modellenbureau Agency
Libellemeent48
Hilversum, 1218 CG Netherlands
T 35 691 5281

Adlinda's Model Agency
Kamp 13-74
Lelystad, 8225 GA Netherlands
T 320 232 213
F 320 232 213

Galucci International Model Agency
Wilhelminasingel 127
Maastricht, 6221 BJ Netherlands
T 43 325 7869
F 43 325 8032

B & T MODEL AGENCY MEPPEL
Biezenveld 54
Meppel, 7943 MD Netherlands
Contact: Alex Boer
T 522 252 788
F 522 252 788
W www.btmodellenburo.nl
E modellen@rendo.dekooi.nl

Max Models
Heemraadssingel 137
Rotterdam, 3022 CO Netherlands
T 10 478 1678
F 10 478 2341

MODEL & TALENT AGENCIES

NEW ZEALAND • COUNTRY CODE: 64

Auckland

62 MODELS & TALENT LTD
St Johns Building, #1 Beresford St City
P.O. Box 33662
Auckland, New Zealand
Contact: Sara Tetro
T 9 377 6262
F 9 376 3329
W www.62models.co.nz
E sara@62models.co.nz

CLYNE MANAGEMENT
26 Airedale Street
Auckland, New Zealand
Contact: Kim Larking
T 9 358 5100
F 9 358 5300
W www.clynemodels.com
E models@clyne.co.nz

JET / GLOBAL MODEL & TALENT AGENCY
P.O. Box 68-746, Newton
Auckland, New Zealand
Contact: Norma McDonald-Tauau
T 9 358 0318
F 9 358 2108
E norma@jetmodels.co.nz

JUNE DOLLY WATKINS MODEL AGENCY
Level 4, 69 Beach Road, Parnell
Auckland, 1 New Zealand
Contact: Sharon Meachen, Director
T 9 379 5474
F 9 373 4072
E jdw@jdwmodels.co.nz

NOVA LTD
P.O. Box 326
Auckland, 1 New Zealand
Contact: Caroline Barley
Physical: Level 2, 79 Anzac Ave, Auckland, 1
T 9 309 9408
F 9 309 8691
W www.nova-models.co.nz
E models@nova-models.co.nz

Christchurch

Clyne Management Inc Exposure Models
160 Tuam Street
Christchurch, New Zealand
T 3 366 0509
F 3 366 0511

Models One
236 High Street, 1st Floor
Christchurch, New Zealand
T 3 377 7101
F 3 377 7181

PORTFOLIO MODEL AGENCY LTD
182 Oxford Terrace, P.O. Box 1133
Christchurch, New Zealand
Contact: Lyn Beazer
T 3 379 9011
F 3 379 6911
W www.modelsnz.co.nz
E portfolio@modelsnz.co.nz

RENAISSANCE MANAGEMENT LTD
190 Hereford Street, Level 4
Kenton Chambers, Suite 408
Christchurch, New Zealand
Contact: Niki Mealings
T 3 963 0718
F 3 963 0719
E renmgmt@clear.net.nz

• • • • • • • • • •

VANITY WALK MODEL & TALENT AGENCY
27 St Andrew Street
Dunedin, New Zealand
Contact: Margaret Farry-Williams
T 3 477 9609
F 3 474 0552
E vanitywalk@xtra.co.nz

THE AGENCIE MANAGEMENT
P.O. Box 6470, Marion Square
60 Ghuznee Str, Level 1
Wellington, New Zealand
Contact: Adelle Kenny
T 4 384 4068
F 4 385 2627
W www.theagencie.com
E enquiries@theagencie.com

Double Happy
25 Majoribanks Street, Mt Victoria 1st Floor
Wellington, New Zealand
T 4 385 8916
F 4 801 5202

MODEL & TALENT AGENCIES

NORWAY • COUNTRY CODE: 47

Kristij Models International
Østre Skostredet 5
Bergen, 5017 Norway
T 5532 1328
F 5532 0980

MODELLHUSET MODEL MANAGEMENT
Vestre Torggate 13
Bergen, 5015 Norway
Contact: Charles
T 5594 4950
F 5594 4951
W www.modellhuset.no
E modell@modellhuset.no

FACE MODELS
Fremskridt 10
Fredrikstad, 1605 Norway
Contact: Kari Dalen
T 6931 3788
F 6931 5705
E kari@face.no

PRESTIGE MODEL AGENCY
Madlamarkv. 118
Hafrsfjord-Stavanger, 4041 Norway
Contact: Inger Løno, Director
T 5155 0391
F 5155 2515
W www.prestige.no
E inger@prestige.no

Oslo

EVERY BODY MODELLER • CASTINGAGENTUR
Kjelsasv, 51D
Oslo, 0488 Norway
Contact: Rene Charles Gustavsen
T 2222 3580
F 2271 0401
E everybody@c2i.net

HEARTBREAK MODEL AGENCY A/S
Sommerrogt 13-15, pb 2307 Solli
Oslo, 0201 Norway
Contact: Björnar Aaslund
T 2254 3900
F 2254 3901
E heartbas@online.no

Mode de Paris
Bygdoy alle 37
Oslo, 0265 Norway
T 2256 1677
F 2256 1677

>>

NORWAY

Team Model & Stylist Management
Baldersgate 18, P.O. Box 3159
Oslo , 0208 Norway
T 2255 8850
F 2243 1554

Elite Modellbyra A/S
Stian Kristensensvei 16
Rykkinn, 1348 Norway
T 6717 2700
F 6717 2710

MODEL & TALENT AGENCIES

PANAMA • COUNTRY CODE: 507

BOB ACTIONS MODELOS
551446 Paitilla, Bikini Plaza
Calle 76, San Francisco
Panama City, Panama
Contact: Guillermo Bobbio / Manuel Aguirre
T 226 5365
F 226 6658
W www.bobactions.com
E models6@panama.c-com.net

MODEL & TALENT AGENCIES

PHILIPPINES • COUNTRY CODE: 63

IDEAL PEOPLE MODEL MANAGEMENT
116 Legazpi Street, P&L Bldg
4th Floor, Legazpi Village
Makati City, Philippines
Contact: Jack B. De Mesa, President
T 2 840 2101
T 2 840 2097
F 2 894 4186
E idealpeople@pacific.net.ph

Image International
15 Abelardo Street, San Lorenzo Village
Makati City, 1223 Philippines
T 2 817 4753
F 2 817 4083

John Robert Powers
195 Salcedo Street, Casmer Bldg, 4th Floor
Metro Manila, 3117 Philippines
T 2 892 9511
F 2 892 7657

MODEL & TALENT AGENCIES

POLAND • COUNTRY CODE: 48

RORES MODELS
P.O. Box 783
Krakow, 30960 Poland
Contact: Zygmuut Fura
T 12 421 6349
T 502 898 930
F 12 421 6349
W www.idm.bcc.pl
E rores@bci.krakow.pl

IMAGE MODEL MANAGEMENT
Ul Libelta 29
Poznan, 61-707 Poland
T 61 851 5483
F 61 855 3484
W www.image-models.com.pl
E image@image-models.com.pl

EASTERN MODELS
Ul Smolna 34/1
Warsaw, 00375 Poland
Contact: Agnieszka Eminowicz
T 22 827 8729
F 22 828 5075
W www.easternmodels.com.pl
E easternmodels@easternmodels.com.pl

LOOK MANAGEMENT
ul. Wilcza 22 / 6A
Warsaw, 00-544 Poland
Contact: Sergiusz Piotrowski, President
T 22 622 4809
T 501 551 953 Mobile
F 22 622 4809
W www.look.pl
E look@pol.pl

Model Plus
Kredytowa 6/1
Warsaw, 00062 Poland
T 22 828 4050
F 22 828 4051

Myskena Studio
Ul. Norwida 19/4
Wroclaw, 50-374 Poland
T 71 328 3268
F 71 328 3268

MODEL & TALENT AGENCIES

PORTUGAL • COUNTRY CODE: 351

A-MODELS
Rua do Mergulhao 3, Cascais
Lisbon, 2750 Portugal
T 9 3336 4014
F 21 484 70 71
E romeo161155@hotmail.com

L'AGENCE, AGENCIA DE MODELOS
Rua Coelho da Rocha, 69- Porta 12
Lisbon, 1300 Portugal
T 1 397 4207
F 1 395 2981

MODEL & TALENT AGENCIES

ROMANIA • COUNTRY CODE: 40

INTERNATIONAL MODELING AGENCY
P.O. Box 27-21, COD 77-550
Bucharest, Romania
Contact: Liviu Miron, President
Representing very famous sport athletes, entertainment artists models, children & talent worldwide
T 1 413 2534 Tel/Fax Only
T 092 223 343 Mobile
W www.domino.ima.kappa.ro
E ima@mail.kappa.ro.
***See Ad This Section.**

M.R.A MODELS AGENCY
49, Dionisie Lupu Street, 3rd Floor, Suite 7
Sector 1, Bucharest, Romania
Contact: Liviu Ionescu, Director
T 1 211 0595
T 1 211 2855
F 1 211 0595

MODEL & TALENT AGENCIES

RUSSIA • COUNTRY CODE: 7

O.M.M. OXANA MODEL MANAGEMENT
119, Sovietskaja Str.
Tambov, 392000 Russia
Contact: Oxana Zoubakova, Managing Director
T 752 472153
F 752 473694
W www.ommrussia.com
E oxana@ommrussia.com

Fast Models
17 Pushkinskaya Street
Vladivostok, 690091 Russia
T 4232 430 730
F 4232 430 963

MODEL & TALENT AGENCIES

SCOTLAND • COUNTRY CODE: 44

GLASGOW MODEL AGENCY
139 Marfield Street
Glasgow, G32 6EZ Scotland
T 141 778 0999
F 141 778 0999

MODEL & TALENT AGENCIES

SINGAPORE • COUNTRY CODE: 65

John Robert Powers
391A Orchard Road, #12-01
Singapore, 238873 Singapore
T 668 6221
F 339 1676

>>

SINGAPORE

MANNEQUIN STUDIO PTE LTD
No 49, Cantonment Road 01-00
Singapore, 089750 Singapore
Contact: Yvonne Tan
T 224 8626
F 224 7163
W www.mannequin.com.sg
E mstudio@mbox3.com.sg

MODEL & TALENT AGENCIES

SLOVAK REPUBLIC • COUNTRY CODE: 421

EXIT MODEL MANAGEMENT
Hlavne namestie 5, 5th Floor
Bratislava, 811 01 Slovak Republic
T 7 544 31 341
T 7 544 31 342
F 7 546 40 711
W www.exitmm.sk
E exitmm@exitmm.sk

FORZA PRODUCTION HOUSE
Bajkalska 25/a
Bratislava 26, 82502 Slovak Republic
T 7 4341 5656
F 7 4341 5521
W www.forza.sk
E forza@isternet.sk

LOOK MODEL MANAGEMENT
Michalska 2
Bratislava, 81101 Slovak Republic
T 7 544 15314
F 7 544 32567

MODEL & TALENT AGENCIES

SLOVENIA • COUNTRY CODE: 386

ADELL'S MODELS
Cesta 1. Maja 68
Hrastnik, 1430 Slovenia
Contact: Mrs. Adela Ackun
T 15 347 601
F 15 072 654

MODEL GROUP
Nazorjeva 2/I
Ljubljana, 1000 Slovenia
T 1 425 2204
T 1 425 2186
F 1 425 2344
W www.model-group.si
E marina.c.masowietsky@model-group.si

MODEL & TALENT AGENCIES

SOUTH AFRICA • COUNTRY CODE: 27

Cape Town

BASE MODEL AGENCY
The Foundry Courtyard, Prestwich Street
Cape Town, 8005 South Africa
Contact: Neal Vincent
T 21 418 2135
F 21 418 2135
W www.faces.co.za
E base@icon.co.za

Boss Models
2nd Floor, CPI House, 220 Loop Street
Cape Town, 8001 South Africa
T 21 424 0224
F 21 423 6967

Elite Model Management
The Studios 112 Buitengracht Street, Suite 508
Cape Town, 8000 South Africa
T 21 422 0004
F 21 422 0007

E-MALE / WOMEN
Suite 324, Sovereign Quay, Somerset Road
Cape Town, 8001 South Africa
Contact: Marsha or Margie
T 21 425 6200
F 21 425 2636
E modelinfo@e-male.co.za

G3 MODEL AGENCY (PTY) LTD
Loft 214, Victoria Junction, Gate 4
Prestwich Street, Green Point
Cape Town, 8001 South Africa
Contact: Anton Gouwsventer
T 21 419 1101
F 21 425 2790
E g3@dockside.co.za

M1 MANAGEMENT
112 Buitengracht Street, 508 The Studios
Cape Town, South Africa
Contact: Erin Sullivan
T 21 422 0004
F 21 422 0007
E models1@mweb.co.za

MAX MODELS
Unit 7, Heritage Square, 100 Shortmarket Street
Cape Town, 8001 South Africa
Contact: Lyn Maxwell
T 21 424 1110
F 21 424 1119
W www.maxmodels.co.za
E info@maxmodels.co.za

The Model Company
28 Wandel Street, Gardens
Cape Town, 8001 South Africa
T 21 462 2461
F 21 461 3869

MODEL TEAM
28 Scott Street, Gardens
Cape Town, 8001 South Africa
Contact: Fiona Craig
T 21 465 0480
T 21 465 0481
F 21 465 6638
E modelt@netactive.co.za

MULLIGAN'S MODEL MANAGEMENT
15 Varneys Road, Green Point
Cape Town, 8051 South Africa
Contact: Carin Kruger
T 21 439 0304
F 21 439 0303
E mulligans@icon.co.za

PUBLIC IMAGE MODELS
The Penthouse, 6th Floor, 24 Burg Street
Cape Town, 8001 South Africa
Contact: Liesel Brukman,
Dylan Stevens, Riaan Kirstein
T 21 426 1416
T 21 423 1610
F 21 426 1619
E pubim@iafrica.com

SCREENFACE MODEL MANAGEMENT AGENCY
120 Buitengracht Street
Cape Town, 8001 South Africa
Contact: Renico Von Rensburg
T 21 423 4065
F 21 423 3643
W www.screenface.co.za
E 2models@screenface.co.za

TOPCO MODELS
9 Bree Street, Touchstone Bldg, 1st Floor
Cape Town, 8001 South Africa
Contact: Linsay Shuttleworth
T 21 419 6162
F 21 419 6165
W www.topcomodels.co
E topco@netactive.co.za

ZERO MODEL MANAGEMENT
12 Greenpoint Mews, 99 Main Road, Greenpoint
Cape Town, 8005 South Africa
Contact: Paul Upton
T 21 434 5744
F 21 434 3077
W www.zeromodels.com
E info@zeromodels.com

G3 MODEL AGENCY (PTY) LTD
1st floor, Hazeldene Hall
13 Junction Avenue, Parktown
Gauteng, 2193 South Africa
Contact: Carl Heunis
T 11 484 3317
F 11 484 3019
E g3models@icon.co.za

Johannesburg

AMM MODELS
173 Oxford Road, Suite 308C, 2nd Floor, Rosebank
Johannesburg, South Africa
Contact: Jenni Vorster, Director
T 11 880 3377
F 11 880 3979
E amm-model@global.co.za

GAPA MODEL AGENCY
Penthouse Suite 1, Thebe House
166 Jan Smuts Avenue
Johannesburg, 2196 South Africa
Contact: Thea Wallner, Owner
T 11 788 4778
F 11 788 1023
E gapa@icon.co.za

HEADS MODEL AGENCY
2nd Floor, "The Mews" Rosebank
Johannesburg, 2196 South Africa
Contact: Monica / Massimo
T 11 442 6020
F 11 442 7306
E niven@icon.co.za

SUPERMODELS
Walbrooke House, 37 Glenhove Road, Melrose Estates
Johannesburg, 2196 South Africa
Contact: Nina Costella, Managing Member
T 11 880 7520
F 11 880 7511
E supermod@global.co.za

TOPCO MODELS
114 Jan Smuts Avenue, Rosebank
Johannesburg, 2193 South Africa
Contact: Patience Muzanenhamo-Lusengo
or Candice Hayward
T 11 880 8660
F 11 880 1813
E personaltouch@pixie.co.za

MODEL & TALENT AGENCIES

SPAIN • COUNTRY CODE: 34

Barcelona

BARBIZON • BARCELONA
Aribau, 117, Ent. 1ª
Barcelona, 08036 Spain
Contact: Peter Sole, President
T 93 414 1317
F 93 209 4032
W www.modelingschools.com/barcelona
E barbizonbcn@jazzfree.com

Elite Models
Av Tibidabo, 56
Barcelona, 08035 Spain
T 93 418 80 99
F 93 211 05 91

FLEMING MODELS
Dr Fleming 13, 4th Floor, 2nd Door
Barcelona, 08017 Spain
Contact: Rachel and Joseph
T 93 209 9902
T 93 209 0802
F 93 209 8088
E agency@flemingmodels.com

Francina
Ronda General Mitre170, ático 2
Barcelona, 08006 Spain
T 93 212 56 26
F 93 418 29 59

GROUP
Pº de Gracia, 67, pral. 1ª
Barcelona, 08008 Spain
T 93 488 2662
F 93 488 0232
W www.groupmodels.com
E info@groupmodels.com

LA AGENCIA MODEL MANAGEMENT
449, Diagonal Avenue
Barcelona, 08036 Spain
Contact: Santiago Lopez-Guix
T 93 444 3000
F 93 444 3001
E la_agencia@seker.es

NATASHA'S MODELS
Avenida Diagonal, 469 6º, 2a
Barcelona, 08036 Spain
Contact: Natasha Gounkevitch
T 93 405 34 35
F 93 439 5456
W www.natashas.com
E natasha-models@natashas.com

Paula's Models
Riera de San Miguel, 55
Barcelona, 08006 Spain
T 93 217 04 94
F 93 217 26 00

SALVADOR MODEL AGENCY
Avda. Diagonal 403
Barcelona, 08008 Spain
Contact: Ana Mills, Women's Division
Montse Gean, Men's Division
T 93 416 00 06
F 93 415 39 50
E salvama@teleline.es

Traffic
Av. Diagonal, 423-425, 2º 1ª
Barcelona, 08036 Spain
T 93 414 0268
F 93 414 6830

• • • • • • • • • •

Olé Model Management
C/ Perez Galdós 23-2P, Santa Cruz de Tenerife
Canary Islands, 38003 Spain
T 922 24 76 56
F 922 24 63 99

This Way
Calle Padre Cueto 14-1º B, Las Palmas
Canary Islands, 35008 Spain
T 928 26 39 55
F 928 27 41 51

Madrid

Avenue
Génova 23, 1st Floor
Madrid, 28004 Spain
T 91 308 29 34
F 91 308 30 03

Delphoss/Mehga Models
Sagasta 4, 2nd Floor
Madrid, 28004 Spain
T 91 521 7373
F 91 532 2951

GROUP
Alcalá 87, 3º
Madrid, 28009 Spain
T 91 431 30 11
F 91 578 12 19
W www.groupmodels.com
E info@groupmodels.com

ISASI Agency & School Models
10 Encarnacion, Bajo Dcha
Madrid, 28013 Spain
T 91 541 60 07
F 91 541 90 43

Magic
Mone-Esquinnza 24-bajo dcha
Madrid, 28010 Spain
T 91 319 2300
F 34 91 310 4841

Maroe Management
Princesa, 31, 7°-3
Madrid, 28008 Spain
T 34 91 548 27 67
F 34 91 541 73 78

Stars Model Agency
Plaza Espana 18, 4°-16
Madrid, 28008 Spain
T 91 541 9690
F 91 542 9657

MODEL & TALENT AGENCIES

SWEDEN • COUNTRY CODE: 46

Avenue Modeller
Östra Hamngatan 50, Box 53020
Göteborg, 40014 Sweden
T 31 774 15 77
F 31 774 15 75

ATOM
Dobelnsgatan 35
Stockholm, 11358 Sweden
T 8 612 0880
F 8 612 0891

MIKAS MODELLKONSULT AB
Ragvaldsgatan 14
Stockholm, 11846 Sweden
Contact: Mika Kjellberg
T 8 578 80000
F 8 641 2145
W www.mias.se

Up! Models
Swedenborgsgatan 7
Stockholm, 11865 Sweden
T 8 462 9585
F 8 462 9588

MODEL & TALENT AGENCIES

SWITZERLAND • COUNTRY CODE: 41

Elite Fribourg
15 Rue des Arsenaux 1700
Fribourg, 1700 Switzerland
T 26 322 3280
F 26 222 4956

NEW FACES MODEL AGENCY
Via Massagno 5
Lugano, 6900 Switzerland
Contact: Franco Taranto, Director
T 91 921 2655
F 91 921 2655
E franco.taranto@smile.ch

MAD COMPANY PEOPLE, MODELS, ARTISTS & ACTORS AGENCY
Am Wasser 158
Zürich, 8049 Switzerland
Contact: Zaruhi Takfor, Director
T 1 342 44 22
F 1 342 44 40
W www.madcompany.com
E info@madcompany.com

MODEL & TALENT AGENCIES

TAIWAN • COUNTRY CODE: 886

FASHION MODEL MANAGEMENT
11F-4, No 230, Sec 2, Shin-Yi Road
Taipei, Taiwan ROC
Contact: Paul Chang
T 2 2394 5258
F 2 2394 5227
W www.fashion-model.com.tw
E fashionn@ms25.hinet.net
***See Ad This Section.**

FMI • FACE MODELS INTERNATIONAL
4F, No 5, Lanes 45, Sec 2, Chung-Shan N Rd.
Taipei, Taiwan ROC
Contact: Emily Chang
T 2 2567 7002
F 2 2567 7004
E fmi58888@ms18.hinet.net

NEW FACE MODEL AGENCY
14F-2, No 230, Sec 2, Shin-Yi Road
Taipei, Taiwan, ROC
Contact: Mr. Paul Chang
T 2 2394 4426
F 2 2341 5651
W www.newface-model.com.tw
E newfaces@ms31.hinet.net
***See Ad This Section.**

>>

PT MODELS
4F, No 171, Sec 4, Pa-Teh Road
Taipei, Taiwan, R.O.C
Contact: Jill Sheu, Managing Director
T 2 2762 7001
F 2 2769 0039
E ptmodels@ms12.hinet.net

QUEENS MODEL AGENCY
9F-4, No 230, Sec 2, Shin-Yi Road
Taipei, Taiwan ROC
Contact: Paul Chang
T 2 2391 3557
F 2 2395 9408
W www.queens-model.com.tw
E queens@ms34.hinet.net
*See Ad This Section.

UNIQUE PREMIER MODEL MANAGEMENT
2F, No. 98, Sec 1, Da An Rd
Taipei, 10551 Taiwan
Contact: Kris Fang
T 2 2773 4668
F 2 2781 1006
W www.uniquepremiermodels.com
E info@uniquepremiermodels.com

MODEL & TALENT AGENCIES

THAILAND • COUNTRY CODE: 66

John Robert Powers
17/F Sitthivorakit Bldg, 5 Soi Pipat, Silom Road
Bangkok, 10500 Thailand
T 2 236 8160
F 2 235 0130

P & N INTERNATIONAL MODEL MANAGEMENT
514/59-60 Thongprasert, Pattanakarn Road,
Suanluang Dist.
Bangkok, 10250 Thailand
Contact: Chin Manasmontri / Khoon Ah
T 2 319 9251
T 2 319 9252
F 2 319 8232

MODEL & TALENT AGENCIES

TURKEY • COUNTRY CODE: 90

Metropolitan-DAME
Fugen sokak, No 5
Istanbul, 80620 Turkey
T 212 282 4192
F 212 282 4150

TOP MODELS OF THE WORLD
Hasanbedrettin Sok 4/7 Hamdi Bey Apt
Istanbul, 81070 Turkey
T 216 355 2119
F 216 363 7136

MODEL & TALENT AGENCIES

URUGUAY • COUNTRY CODE: 598

VALENTINO BOOKINGS INTERNATIONAL
Colon 1476, Ap 502
Montevideo, CP 11000 Uruguay
Contact: Carlos Camara, Director
T 2 915 1277
F 2 915 2867
W www.elcanal.com/valentino
E valentino.bookings@correoweb.com

MODEL & TALENT AGENCIES

VENEZUELA • COUNTRY CODE: 58

Bookings International Model Agency
Av Caurimare, Colinas de Bella Monte Qta 284
Caracas, 1042 Venezuela
T 52 751 2013
F 2 751 2446

MODEL & TALENT AGENCIES

YUGOSLAVIA • COUNTRY CODE: 381

LOOK MODEL MANAGEMENT
Admirala Geprata 14
Belgrade, 11000 Yugoslavia
T 11 361 72 49
F 11 361 72 49
E look@eunet.yu

Notes

GENERAL INDEX

ADVERTISERS INDEX

Thank You to all our advertisers
for your continued support.

The times in the following cities and countries are it is 12:00 noon (Eastern Standard Time) in New York City. Listing in italics are the times the next calendar day.

Anchorage	8:00 am
Argentina	2:00 pm
Australia (Perth)	1:00 am
Austria	6:00 pm
Bahamas	12:00 noon
Belgium	6:00 pm
Bermuda	1:00 pm
Brazil	2:00 pm
Canada (Toronto)	12:00 noon
Chicago	11:00 am
Chile	1:00 pm
China	1:00 am
Colombia	12:00 noon
Costa Rica	11:00 am
Denmark	6:00 pm
Denver	10:00 am
Detroit	12:00 noon
Dominican Republic	12:00 am
Egypt	7:00 pm
England	5:00 pm
Finland	7:00 pm
France	6:00 pm
Germany	6:00 pm
Greece	7:00 pm
Guam	3:00 am
Hong Kong	1:00 am
Houston	11:00 am
Hungary	6:00 pm
India	10:30 pm
Indonesia	12:00 am
Ireland	5:00 pm
Israel	7:00 pm
Italy	6:00 pm
Jamaica	11:00 am
Japan	2:00 am
Korea	2:00 am
Los Angeles	9:00 am
Mexico (Mexico City)	11:00 am
Miami	12:00 noon
Netherlands	6:00 pm
New Zealand	5:00 am
Norway	6:00 pm
Pakistan	10:00 am
Peru	12:00 noon
Phillipines	1:00 am
Poland	6:00 pm
Portugal (mainland)	6:00 pm
Puerto Rico	1:00 pm
Russia (Moscow)	8:00 pm
Singapore	1:00 am
South Africa	7:00 pm
Spain	6:00 pm
Sri Lanka	10:30 pm
Switzerland	6:00 pm
Thailand	12:00 am
Uruguay	2:00 pm
Venezuela	1:00 pm
West Indes	1:00 pm
Zaire	6:00 pm